6

**W9-ADH-211**

# WIN
## THE
# SUGAR
# WAR

# WIN
## THE
# SUGAR
# WAR

## 100 Real-Life Stories of Conquering Cravings—And Pounds

# HOLLY McCORD, R.D.
NUTRITION EDITOR, *PREVENTION* MAGAZINE

RODALE

© 2002 by Rodale Inc.

Cover photograph of Holly McCord by Hilmar
Profile photos courtesy of participants

Printed in the United States of America

Interior design by Christina Gaugler and Carol Angstadt
Cover design by Carol Angstadt
Series cover design by Andrew Newman

ISBN 1–57954–530–0

**Distributed to the book trade by St. Martin's Press**

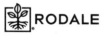

WE **INSPIRE** AND **ENABLE** PEOPLE TO IMPROVE
THEIR LIVES AND THE WORLD AROUND THEM

# CONTENTS

# ACKNOWLEDGMENTS

A s a magazine editor, I know that behind every byline is a team of gifted individuals who work tirelessly to ensure that every sentence in an article is accurate, thoughtful, and compelling. The same is true for this book.

I'm profoundly grateful to all those who contributed to *Win the Sugar War*, beginning with the 100 women and men who volunteered to share their stories with us—and with you. Each one of these people is an inspiration. Without them, this book would not exist.

Many others have played a part in transforming *Win the Sugar War* from a germ of an idea into 256 pages of engaging, entertaining, empowering prose. For their time and talents, I want to recognize and thank Tami Booth, Susan Berg, Jean Rogers, Elizabeth Shimer, Winnie Yu, Laura Catalano, Linda Formichelli, W. Eric Martin, Lynn Reynolds Parks, Sandi Lloyd, Jennifer Goldsmith, Lori Davis, Barb Fexa, Lynn Goldstein, Jennifer Kowalak, Jan McLeod, Elizabeth Price, Gwen Taylor, Lucille Uhlman, Lisa Vroman, Teresa Yeykal, Nancy Zelko, Madeleine Adams, Jane Sherman, Marilyn Hauptly, Darlene Schneck, Carol Angstadt, Chris Gaugler, Bethany Bodder, Jodi Schaffer, and Julie Kehs Minnix.

I also want to express my appreciation to my colleagues in the Rodale Women's Health Group for their ongoing support of *Win the Sugar War*. Special thanks go to Catherine Cassidy, Sarah Robertson, Amy Rhodes, Leslie Schneider, Dana Bacher, Lisa Dolin, Lorraine Rodriguez, Cindy Ratzlaff, and Mary Lengle.

# INTRODUCTION

## *ARE YOU READY TO WIN THE SUGAR WAR?*

Because I'm a registered dietitian, most people expect me to have some sort of ingrained resistance to sweets. After all, I—of all people—should understand the potential consequences of eating too much sugar.

But just try reminding me of that when I'm holed up in a hotel room with a mini-bar, and its stash of overpriced candy bars, within arm's reach. On more than a few occasions, especially when I couldn't sleep, I've broken down and shelled out $5 or $6 for one Snickers bar or bag of M&M's.

The fact is, I love sweet things. I'd eat a pint of ice cream or a bag of Pepperidge Farm Milanos every night, if only I could avoid the repercussions. I weaken more often than I like to admit.

In other words, I'm no different than you and everyone else who is at the mercy of a ravenous sweet tooth. I'm tempted, I indulge, I feel guilty, I resolve to be stronger the next time. Then the next time comes . . . and how can I resist?

The dietitian in me knows that an occasional sweet won't do any harm. It's eating too much sugar that can contribute to weight gain—plus fatigue, nutrient deficiencies, insulin resistance, and assorted other health concerns. And these days, sweets are everywhere, so it's way too easy to overindulge.

What's a health-conscious sugar aficionado to do?

For answers, I sought out the real experts—100 women and men who have come up with some very ingenious ways of reining in their sugar consumption. Their stories are the heart and soul of *Win the Sugar War*.

These people cited all sorts of reasons for wanting to cut back on sweets. Some had serious health problems and were under doctors' orders to reduce their sugar intake. Others realized that their cravings for cookies and candy bars were being driven by emotional upheaval or uncontrolled stress. Many noticed that their clothes fit too snugly and blamed sugar for the extra pounds.

Whatever their motivation, all of these people mustered the willpower to wean themselves off sweets. Perhaps most amazing to me, once they did it, they never went back. Most have been sugar-free for years, even decades.

So read their stories and sample their Winning Actions, the strategies that enabled them to conquer their sweet cravings once and for all. Of course, not every Winning Action will appeal to every person. The beauty of this book is that you have *choices*. Try the strategies that best suit your needs and lifestyle and discard those that don't produce the results you expect. In this way, you'll create your very own, customized plan for winning the sugar war.

Before jumping into the personal stories, be sure to read through the three introductory chapters. They provide some fascinating background on why we humans crave sweets (it's in our genes!), where we get most of our sugar (sodas are the number one source), and how overindulging undermines our health (as mentioned earlier, weight gain is just one of the effects). Especially helpful are the 10 Tools for Living Sugar-Free (page 1), which lay the foundation for subduing even the most formidable sweet tooth.

To get a handle on your personal sugar intake, follow the simple self-tests in "Crossing the 'Too-Much' Threshold" on page 25. And don't forget to check out the chart on page 234, which offers the sugar content of a sampling of foods within the five major categories of sweets. Did you know that a slice of pumpkin pie has more sugar than a glazed doughnut, or that a serving of granola is sweeter than a serving of Kellogg's Frosted Flakes? It surprised me, too!

That brings me to a couple of important points. First, if you want to cut back on sugar, your best bet is to focus on *added* sugars—the kinds found in many prepared and packaged foods, including those mentioned above. Added sugars deliver lots of extra calories but nothing in the way of nutrition. Just giving up your morning toaster pastry or your lunchtime cola can make a substantial dent in your sugar and calorie intake—and leave room for more nutritious food choices.

Second, you don't need to swear off sugar completely to notice positive changes in your health, including in your waistline. You will meet people in this book who felt that they had to oust every last granule of sweetness from their diets if they wanted to succeed. They have my profound admiration, because frankly, I just couldn't do it. I enjoy sweets too much. Most nutrition experts agree that as long as we keep our sugar consumption moderate, we won't do ourselves any harm.

So we *can* have our cake—or cola or candy bar—and eat it, too. We just can't eat too much. Choose your indulgences carefully, and you'll discover that even though your diet may be a little less sugary, your life is no less sweet.

# 10 Tools
# for Living
# Sugar-Free

S o you've decided to break free from chocolate, to end your love affair with éclairs, to cancel your regular 8 P.M. date with a bowl of ice cream. Good for you! You've taken a big step toward winning the sugar war. After all, recognizing that you eat too many sweets is half the battle. And as you'll learn from the inspirational real-life stories later in this book, actually reducing your sugar consumption doesn't have to be a battle at all. You just need the will to start and the motivation and means to stay on track.

To that end, the following 10 tools can help you achieve a less sugar-dependent—though no less sweet—existence. You may feel that some tools are more relevant to your particular situation than others. That's fine. Pick and choose as you wish—though do read all of them. Together they provide a "big picture" perspective that just might convince you that you *can* take charge of an insatiable sweet tooth.

## Tool #1: Stop and Think Before You Eat

You nervously nibble on Jujubes while watching a suspenseful movie, and before you know it, you reach into the box and feel the bottom. Or you groggily sprinkle teaspoon after teaspoon of sugar onto your morning bowl of cereal until it seems like it should be sweet enough. Yes, mindlessly eating sugar is that easy—and all of us do it from time to time.

In order to reduce the amount of sugar in your diet, you've got to pay attention to what you're putting into your mouth. Some people keep a "food diary" just for this purpose, writing down what they eat and when—and sometimes even why. If that doesn't appeal to you, then make a point of pausing and contemplating every food choice. For example, if you're dining out with friends and everyone else orders a pastry of some sort for dessert, don't just follow suit. Instead, think about what you ate the rest of the day. If you had a Danish and Coke for breakfast, you should probably abstain.

The same is true when you're cooking. You don't need to follow recipes to the letter, especially if they call for added sugar. In fact, you can gradually reduce the amount of sugar called for in recipes by one-third—and you just may prefer the slightly less sweet taste. You can get by with ½ cup of sugar per cup of flour in cakes, 1 teaspoon of sugar per cup of flour in yeast breads, and 1 tablespoon of sugar per cup of flour in muffins and quick breads. You can also replace some of the sugar with spices. Nutmeg, ginger, cardamom, mace, and cinnamon make wonderful natural sweeteners.

And be extra wary about using sugary condiments on otherwise healthy foods. If you're in the habit of topping your toast with 2 tablespoons of a fruit preserve, try cutting back to 1 tablespoon—

you'll save 48 calories and 10 grams of sugar. Likewise, instead of saturating your pancakes with syrup, pour a small puddle of syrup onto your plate and dip in each forkful of pancake. You'll be better able to monitor the amount of syrup you've eaten.

Once you've measured out the proper amount of the condiment of your choice, don't set the rest on the table. Put it away. Then if you want more, you've got to go get it—and you just may decide you don't want it after all.

## Tool #2: Figure Out What's Driving Your Cravings

Just when you think you have the upper hand on your sugar intake, along comes a craving to test your resolve. You *know* you don't really need that sweet, but your tongue and your stomach have other ideas. Before you know it, your hand is in the cookie jar.

Sugar cravings are strong, immediate, and sometimes very specific—you *need* that chocolate cupcake with peanut butter icing from the bakery down the street. The best way to defeat a craving is to get to its source. More likely than not, it has some underlying physical or psychological explanation.

Perhaps you're not getting enough of the nutrients your body needs. Give yourself a refresher course on the Food Guide Pyramid and its recommended daily servings of fruits (2 to 4), veggies (3 to 5), grains (6 to 11), and protein (2 to 3 dairy, plus 2 to 3 from your choice of meat, poultry, fish, and beans). These foods can shore up your supply of key vitamins and minerals, which may make your cravings subside.

Then again, maybe you're not eating often enough. Go a few hours without food and you're ready to devour anything in sight, especially something sugary. Eating mini-meals throughout the day can keep your blood sugar stable and your cravings at bay.

Cravings could mean that your body has become dependent on sugar for a quick energy boost. Sweet foods initially give you a surge of stimulation and help you concentrate, but invariably, those good feelings are followed by an equally fast crash.

Force of habit can drive cravings, too. When you were growing up, your mom always served dessert after dinner, so now your taste buds are ready and waiting for a few cookies once the dishes are cleared away.

Of course, PMS is well-known for pushing women toward the candy aisle. That's because the body's feel-good hormones fall off right before menstruation. Women try to compensate by seeking out sweet, decadent foods.

Cravings can even result from dehydration. In that case, you can wash them away by drinking more water. To stay adequately hydrated, you need at least eight 8-ounce glasses of water a day.

The bottom line: If cravings are pushing you to eat more sugar than you know you should, think about what's behind them. Simply acknowledging the cause—and taking appropriate preemptive action—may switch off your desire for sweets.

## Tool #3: Focus on the Big Five

We get most of our sugar from foods in five key categories: soda, sweetened baked goods, candy, ice cream, and sweetened fruit drinks.

Of these, soda reigns as king of the Big Five. That's no surprise. Many of us have the mind-set that soda "doesn't count" as a source of sugar and calories, since it's a liquid. Make no mistake: It does count. A 20-ounce serving of nondiet soda supplies 85 grams of sugar.

Next among the Big Five is candy, followed by sweetened baked goods, which include sugary cereals, muffins, cakes, and all other sweets that once saw the inside of an oven. You probably know that cookies and cakes have more than modest amounts of sugar, but cereals can be deceiving. Raisin Bran sounds healthy, and in some respects, it is. But it can be loaded with sugar.

Ice cream ranks fourth on the list of top sugar sources. Sweetened fruit drinks may be last, but they're not to be disregarded. Some fruit drinks and canned teas deliver 20 to 30 grams of sugar in a 1-cup serving.

## Tool #4: Think "Moderation" Rather Than Elimination

If you're like the average American, you eat 16 to 20 teaspoons (64 to 80 grams) of sugar a day—twice the amount experts recommend if you want to maintain good health. But in *moderation*, sugar is not necessarily bad.

You will not get fat just because you eat sweets. Too much of *any* food is what leads to extra pounds. Small amounts of sugar are fine, particularly if you're physically active. In fact, trying to completely eliminate sugar may make you more likely to overindulge, because you'll break down and eat everything sweet in sight.

A good rule to follow is to get no more than 10 percent of your daily calories from added sugar. For most adults, this equals about 50 grams a day. To give you an idea of how little sugar this is: If you were to consume one small glass of Kool-Aid and a package of Hostess Devil's Food Twinkies, you'd exceed your 50-gram limit.

To stay within your sugar quota, eat no more than one sweet treat a day and steer clear of all sugar-sweetened beverages. And before you eat your treat, fill up on vegetables or lean proteins, so you're less likely to want more sugar.

And don't let natural sugars (like honey, molasses, and brown sugar) fool you into thinking they're better for you. Both table sugar and natural sugars have the same negative health effects, raising blood sugar and supplying empty calories instead of important nutrients. So remember that natural sugars count toward your 10 percent cap.

## Tool #5: Read Nutrition Labels Religiously

As you peruse the supermarket aisles, you can use labels to size up the sugar content of foods. But you need to know what to look for. Sugar may be listed in two separate places: the Nutrition Facts and the ingredients list. The Nutrition Facts specifies the amount of sugar in a serving. The ingredients list identifies added sugars by name.

Just because a label says 10 grams of sugar doesn't mean that food should be banished from your grocery cart. Some foods—like milk, beans, and fruits—naturally contain sugars that don't appear in the ingredients list. Still, they count toward the amount of sugar in the Nutrition Facts.

The ingredients appear in descending order by weight (meaning from highest to lowest). The closer an ingredient is to the start of the list, the more of it is in the food. If you see two or more sugars near the top spot, you may want to leave that food on the supermarket shelf.

Sugars go by many names. Be on the lookout for honey, brown sugar, raw sugar, turbinado sugar, dextrose, maltose, high-fructose corn syrup, molasses, dextrin, invert sugar, caramel, corn sweetener, and confectioner's sugar, among others.

And don't fall for tricks of the food industry trade. Instead of adding a large amount of one type of sugar, which would place it near the beginning of the ingredients list, some manufacturers use smaller amounts of several forms of sugar so they appear farther down the list. For example, Quaker Toasted Oatmeal Honey Nut cereal contains sugar, molasses, brown sugar, honey, and corn syrup solids—all sugars.

Be careful with low-fat and nonfat foods, too. You may get

more sugar in place of the fat. Some brands of low-fat and nonfat ice cream contain 40 or more grams of sugar per 1-cup serving.

## Tool #6: Find Satisfying Alternatives to Sweets

When your sweet tooth speaks up, you would swear that nothing but a sweet could quiet it. But you may be surprised. Many people have found satisfying alternatives to sweets, and so can you.

With a little time, you can learn to enjoy the naturally sweet taste of fruits, vegetables, and other whole foods. Instead of sweetened yogurt, try plain yogurt with strawberries and bananas. Craving a cinnamon bun for breakfast? Eat a cinnamon raisin bagel with nonfat cream cheese or a toaster waffle with fresh fruit. A homemade smoothie with real fruit and fruit juice can be just as creamy and flavorful as a milk shake. Other good substitutes for sugar-laden treats include frozen bananas, apple slices with peanut butter, and graham crackers topped with applesauce.

Instead of soda, drink water or unsweetened iced tea. Both are more thirst-quenching and satisfying anyway. Citrus staves off cravings for some people, so if you get the urge to eat something sweet, reach for a grapefruit, orange, or tangerine or squeeze some lemon into a glass of water.

Of course, you can buy artificially sweetened versions of almost all your favorite sugary foods. Calorie-free sweeteners like saccharin and aspartame can mimic sugar in treats like baked goods, breakfast cereals, and diet soda. If you usually drink three colas a day and you switch to diet, you'll save 453 calories and 150 grams of sugar.

## Tool #7: Lift Your Mood without Food

If you reach for cookies and candy to feel good or maintain an already good mood, you're not alone. Most of us eat for emotional reasons, at least once in a while.

Maybe you quarreled with your spouse, or you had a stressful day on the job, or you just feel bored. You deserve some cheering up, but sweets are not the way to do it.

Instead, engage in a nonfood activity that lifts your spirits and eliminates boredom or gloominess. For example, try taking a brisk walk—exercise raises levels of endorphins, the mood-enhancing brain chemicals that you're attempting to stimulate with sugar. Laughter has the same effect on endorphins, so watch a funny movie or television show or call a friend who has a knack for telling jokes.

Curl up with a sewing project or a good book. Put on your favorite CD and dance—you'll burn some calories *and* feel good. Dig around in your garden. Paint a picture. Do anything that will distract you from thoughts of a hot-fudge sundae.

Make a list of chores you've been meaning to accomplish and physical activities you enjoy. Each time you feel a mood-driven craving coming on, choose an item from your list. Chances are you'll get so caught up in what you're doing that you'll forget you wanted something sweet in the first place.

## Tool #8: Remember *Why* You Want to Change

In the throes of a craving, you can easily rationalize that you don't need to cut back on sugar after all. But a quick reminder of sugar's not-so-sweet side effects can stop you from opening that chocolate bar.

For one, sugar makes you tired. When you eat a doughnut or a piece of cake, you get a surge of energy. But it doesn't last—and it can leave you feeling even more fatigued than before. Giving up some sugar will get you off the energy roller coaster.

It can also keep you looking young. A recent study has linked excessive sugar consumption with the formation of wrinkles. Think about that the next time you're spooning your way through a pint of ice cream.

That's not all. Sugar can rob you of sleep and put you at greater risk for nutrient deficiencies. Plus, it may stimulate your appetite for all foods, making weight loss much more difficult.

Of course, any discussion of sugar wouldn't be complete without mentioning cavities. The acid coating left on your teeth by sugary foods can destroy the enamel and lead to decay. Now there's a mental image that can easily switch off your desire for sweets!

All this is just the beginning. Over the long term, excessive sugar consumption can raise your risk for a host of health problems, including diabetes, heart disease, high blood pressure, and colon and rectal cancers. Ask yourself: Is sugar really worth it?

## Tool #9: See Results in Places Other Than the Scale

Cut out some sugar and you're going to see some changes in yourself that you're guaranteed to love.

First and foremost, if you've been carrying around a few unwanted pounds, they just might disappear. Don't go by the number on the bathroom scale alone; notice if your clothes feel looser, too. They should. That's because you're eliminating not just the sugar calories but also the fat calories that are often packed into sugary foods like doughnuts, ice cream, cake, and chocolate.

Beyond looking better, you'll feel better, physically and emotionally. If you've been bothered by ailments like allergies, insomnia, and heart palpitations, your symptoms may subside. You may also have a clearer complexion and fewer colds and headaches.

You'll feel more energetic, because you're eating fewer sweets and more of the nutrient-dense foods that help fend off fatigue. Your energy level will be more constant and sustained, which is more healthful than the short-term nervous jitters brought on by sugar.

Emotionally, you'll be free of the mood swings sometimes caused by sugary foods. And you'll feel more powerful and in control, because you're no longer trapped in sugar's clutches.

## Tool #10: Celebrate Every Victory, No Matter How Small

As much as you want to win the sugar war, you need to be realistic and not expect too much too soon. Focus on making small, gradual changes as you work toward reducing your sugar consumption.

Most important, think positively. If you're going to wean yourself from sweets, you've got to believe you can do it.

Set a goal for yourself—say, to stop choosing sweets for snacks—then break it down into manageable steps. One by one, incorporate each step into your lifestyle. You may want to track your progress in a journal. If that's not your style, try posting reminders in places where you're most likely to be tempted by sugar cravings.

When you successfully complete a step, do something nice for yourself. For example, suppose that instead of using your afternoon break to grab a candy bar from the vending machine, you go outside for a walk. On your way back to the office, stop to buy some flowers for your desk. If you get through the supermarket's frozen food section without putting any ice cream into your cart, reward yourself with the latest issue of your favorite magazine. If you resist ordering a piece of pie at dinner, head for the video store afterward to pick up that movie you've been wanting to see.

Naturally, reaching a bigger goal calls for a bigger splurge. If you go an entire week without snacking on sweets, schedule a half-day off for an afternoon of pampering at a nearby day spa or a round of golf. Even plan a weekend getaway, if your budget allows. Do what makes you feel good to celebrate your pending independence from sugar. You deserve it!

# What Causes Those Cravings?

**D**oughnuts appear in the break room at work. Why not have one? It will taste great with the coffee. The teenager next door sells candy to support her softball team. Hey, it's for a good cause. The local supermarket offers free samples of a new frozen yogurt. What the heck—it's free!

We come up with any excuse to eat sweets. And it's no wonder we let our sweet teeth guide us—nature intended it that way. "Back in the primitive days, eating foods that tasted sweet was a good idea, because it meant they were probably ripe and safe to consume," says Hillary Wright, R.D., nutrition coordinator for Harvard Vanguard Medical Associates in Boston.

This desire for sweetness has stayed with us. We eat more sugar than ever before. We want sugar so badly that some of us have become addicted. For the problem cravers among us, scientists are working on a "sugar patch" to make quitting sweets a bit easier.

And the sweets industry is booming. In 1999, cookies accounted for 48.4 percent of baked goods sales. By 2004, sales of packaged sweet foods are expected to exceed $12.2 billion.

But today, unlike in primitive times, eating sugar at every opportunity hurts our health. For one thing, all this sugar is making us fat. According to the National Institutes of Health, 55 percent of the adult population is overweight, and 22 percent is obese.

Besides weight gain, other health problems are linked to sugar overindulgence. Eating too much can lead to dental cavities, fatigue, high blood pressure, and diabetes, just to name a few causes for concern.

If you consider yourself a slave to sweets, it's time you regained your independence. To do this, you must first understand sugar—what it is, where it's found, and why we humans crave it so much.

## What Is Sugar?

Chemically speaking, sugar and white bread are the same thing: carbohydrates that are made up of carbon, hydrogen, and oxygen molecules. But the number and arrangement of those molecules differ.

Many of the sugars that occur in foods are made from combinations of simple sugars, or monosaccharides. For example, sucrose—white table sugar—is glucose paired with fructose, while lactose—the sugar in milk—consists of glucose and galactose.

Once inside your body, sugars are broken down into their simple sugar components. These simple sugars are converted to glucose, which is used for energy by your body's cells.

While your body needs sugar to function, if you're like most people, you're probably getting much more than you should. Your best bet is to stick with naturally occurring sugars because they're found in foods that provide vitamins, minerals, and other nutrients that keep you healthy. For instance, milk supplies not just lactose but also calcium, riboflavin, and protein, and it helps reduce the risk of osteoporosis. Oranges contain vitamin C, folate, and fiber along with fructose; they may help reduce the risk of cancer and heart disease.

On the other hand, white table sugar and the sugars added to processed foods deliver nothing but empty calories, and too much can take a real toll on your health. If you eat these sugars at all, make sure it's in moderation.

## How Much Sugar Do We Eat?

The fact is, in terms of sugar consumption, most of us are well beyond moderation. The average American eats the equivalent of 20 teaspoons of added sugar a day. (Added sugars hide behind a number of names on food labels, including high-fructose corn syrup, invert sugar, dextrose, maltose, glucose, molasses, caramel, barley malt, crystalline fructose, and honey.) At 16 calories per teaspoon, that's 320 calories—16 to 20 percent of our total calorie intake and twice as much as we should get in a day.

The United States Department of Agriculture recommends getting no more than 6 to 10 percent of our daily calories from added sugars. For a 1,600-calorie-a-day diet, that translates to 6 teaspoons or 24 grams of sugar; for 2,000 calories, 10 teaspoons or 40 grams; and for 2,200 calories, 12 teaspoons or 48 grams. Keep in mind, these numbers are conservative. Many of us seriously underestimate our consumption of sweets.

The fat-free craze of the 1990s is largely to blame for our increasing sugar intake. In the early nineties, we all ran from fat—the root of all evil, diet-related health problems, or so we thought. What we didn't realize then is that manufacturers added gobs of sugar to keep consumers' taste buds interested in their "guilt-free" products.

But we should have been feeling guilty, because fat-free isn't so innocent after all. Low-fat and fat-free products sometimes contain more sugar than their full-fat alternatives. For example, a serving of reduced-fat SnackWell's Chocolate Sandwich Cookies with Chocolate Cream contains 11 grams of sugar. A serving of full-fat Archway Dutch Cocoa Cookies contains 8 grams of sugar.

"A recent dietary survey showed that people eat less fat than they did 10 years ago, but on average, they consume 211 more *calories* a day, which is proof that these calories are coming from other sources," says Wright.

The popular myth that natural added sugars are more healthful than refined sugars may be fueling our gluttony. We think: Hey, this honey provides some good stuff *and* it tastes good, so I might as well have some more. "But the healthfulness of honey is so negligible it's not even worth counting," says Therese Franzese, R.D., director of nutrition at the Peninsula Spa and Health Club in New York City. The same goes for brown sugar, raw sugar, corn syrup, maple syrup, and other seemingly healthier sugars. The bottom line is they all contain empty calories. They all add pounds.

## Where Do We Get Our Sugar?

Sugar lurks where we least expect it, like in ketchup and barbecue sauce. "Often, the amount of sugar already present in foods far exceeds the amount we spoon onto foods," says Harry Preuss, M.D., professor of physiology at Georgetown University School of Medicine in Washington, D.C.

Ironically, levels are sometimes lower in foods we avoid because we think they're too sweet. For example, a serving of orange sherbet contains 24 grams of sugar, while a serving of vanilla ice cream has only 20 grams. A serving of fruit drink can have more sugar than a serving of ice cream—32 grams in 8 ounces of Minute Maid Fruit Punch, compared with 30 grams in ½ cup of Ben & Jerry's Chocolate Fudge Brownie ice cream. And low-fat granola packs more sugar than Kellogg's Frosted Flakes.

Favorite sugary foods vary based on age and sex. Women ages 18 to 54 get most of their sugar from soft drinks, as do men 18 to 65. Women 55 and up prefer sweetened baked goods, like cookies and cakes. Men switch from soda to sweetened baked goods as their favorite after age 65.

But overall, we get most of our sugar from the following five food categories.

**Nondiet soda.** The thought of downing 9 to 11 teaspoons of straight table sugar is repulsive, yet soda delivers even more sugar than that—between 8 and 16 teaspoons in one 20-ounce bottle. Soda pop makes up one-third of our intake of added sugars. Half of all American adults and most adolescents drink at least one nondiet soda a day.

"Soda is pure sugar, and it provides nothing in the way of nutrition," says Wright. A can of Coke serves up 150 calories from sugar—that's 100 percent of your recommended sugar intake for the whole day. "Many people don't consider the calories they drink—only the ones they chew," says Wright. But beverages are often the biggest sugar suppliers.

And it's not only the sugar in soda that's harmful. Often, people who choose soft drinks over milk or other dairy products don't get enough calcium. And that can contribute to osteoporosis, a disease characterized by fragile and broken bones.

**Candy.** Seventeen percent of the sugar we eat comes from

candy. Per serving, most candies come close to or exceed the recommended 6 to 10 teaspoons per day. For example, a serving of Strawberry Twizzlers has 6.5 teaspoons of sugar, a 1.69-ounce package of M&M's has 7.7 teaspoons, a Butterfinger bar has 7.2 teaspoons, and a package of Skittles has 7.8 teaspoons.

As with baked goods, low-fat or fat-free candy often has more sugar than candies containing fat, like chocolate. "I have one client who would probably lose those last 5 pounds, but she can't give up her candy—and it's fat-free candy, like Tootsie Rolls and jelly beans," says Franzese.

**Sweet baked goods.** Cookies, cakes, muffins, and other sweetened grain-based foods closely follow candy in the big-five ranks, comprising 16 percent of our sugar intake. Sugary cereals also fall into this category. Typically, just one serving of sweetened grains uses up—or exceeds—our allotted 6 to 10 teaspoons. Two Hostess Low-Fat Chocolate Cupcakes have 9.5 teaspoons of sugar, a serving of Little Debbie Oatmeal Raisin Cookies has 7.2 teaspoons, and Kellogg's Cocoa Krispies cereal has 3.5 teaspoons.

**Ice cream.** If you still feel a twinge of excitement when you hear that familiar ice cream truck bell at the beach, you're not alone. Ice cream is the fourth most popular sugar supplier, and it makes up 10 percent of our sugar consumption. But it's not much better than the baked goods. Breyers Natural Vanilla has 3.8 teaspoons per half-cup serving, and Häagen-Dazs Cookie Dough Chip has 4.8 teaspoons.

**Fruit drinks and sweetened iced tea.** If you think a fruit drink is a better choice than soda, think again. The last of the big five, sweetened beverages comprise 8 percent of our sugar intake. A 20-ounce Fruitopia has 19.2 teaspoons of sugar, at least 9 *more* than a 20-ounce Coke. Eight ounces of Hawaiian Fruit Punch contains 7.5 teaspoons of sugar, 1.5 more than the same amount of 7UP. Whatever you choose, just one bottle or can puts you over the 6- to 10-teaspoon limit.

## Why Do We Desire Sugar?

Among all sweets, chocolate has the distinction of being the most craved food in North America. One classic 1991 study revealed that chocolate constitutes nearly half of all food cravings. Most choco-holics probably don't keep unsweetened baking chocolate among the stash in their desks, so sugar is no doubt a large part of choco-late's seduction.

No one knows for sure why we desire sugar. "There's so much information and misinformation that they almost cancel each other out," says Carolyn Dean, M.D., N.D., a medical writer and media consultant in City Island, New York, and author of *Dr. Carolyn Dean's Natural Prescriptions for Common Ailments.*

Here are some of the most popular theories concerning why some of us find sugar so irresistible.

**Sugar is fuel on reserve.** "In terms of evolution, sweet is neces-sary because it builds energy and provides nourishment when we're sick or hurt," says Dr. Dean. In prehistoric days, when we still for-aged for food, honey was a real find—a chance to stock up on some yummy calories.

The problem is that honey is no longer the gold mine it was prehistorically—today, we're surrounded by sugary foods. "When I was a kid, we had treats once a week. But now that sweets are so readily available, once a week has become several times a day for this generation of kids," says Dr. Dean. "No one is reminding people that too much sugar is not good."

**Old habits die hard.** "I think environment—what children are exposed to when they're young—plays a tremendous role in sugar consumption later in life," says Susan Kleiner, Ph.D., R.D., author of *Power Eating* and owner of High Performance Nutrition in Mercer Island, Washington. For example, if your parents always gave you juice or soda instead of water when you were thirsty, you may not find water particularly tasty or thirst quenching as an adult. And if you grew up with ice cream after every dinner, switching to fruit or abstaining from dessert altogether can be tough.

"On the flip side, it could be that you were deprived of sweets growing up, and now you can't get enough as an adult," adds Franca Alphin, R.D., clinical associate with the department of community and family medicine at Duke University in Durham, North Carolina.

**Some of us have a saber sweet tooth.** Your genes could also be the culprit. "I raised my daughters the same way, and one is a candy junkie, while the other couldn't care less about sweets. I think something natural is going on there," says Dr. Kleiner. It could be a difference in taste buds or a difference in the amount of flavor needed to enjoy food, she says.

In two recent preliminary studies, researchers found that sweet-sensitive mice and sweet-insensitive mice had two distinct versions of the area of DNA responsible for detecting sweetness. The researchers speculate that the same genetic variations may exist in humans.

Another driving factor behind our desire for sweets may be levels of leptin, the hormone that regulates appetite and tells us we're full. When Japanese researchers studied a group of mice, they found that the lower the leptin, the more intense the cravings for sweets, and vice versa. In the presence of high leptin levels, the tongue is less sensitive to the taste of sugar.

**Our lifestyles need some work.** Missing meals or eating the wrong foods can interfere with hormonal regulations and lead to cravings. And fatigue caused by lack of exercise can make us seek out a quick sugary boost.

"Sugar cravings can be a product of poor lifestyle—lack of exercise and carbohydrate overload," says Charles Mabray, M.D., an obstetrician/gynecologist practicing in Victoria, Texas. People skip breakfast, eat a really bad lunch, and don't work out, and then they wonder why they have this huge hunger for chocolate at 3 o'clock.

It may also be time to hit the hobby shop. When the mind isn't occupied, it tends to drift toward food, particularly sweets. "You don't know what to do with yourself, so you say, 'Let's eat . . . let's do *something*,'" says Dr. Preuss.

**We're stressed.** There is a definite connection between stress and sugar cravings, but whether that connection is physiological or psychological is under debate. One physiological theory is that during stress, when the adrenal glands pump out adrenaline and cortisol (the stress hormones), adrenaline causes the heart rate to increase and the liver to supply glucose—"fuel for fight or flight," says Dr. Dean. Then cortisol encourages you to replenish your body's fuel supply by increasing your appetite. Your body thinks it needs sugar for physical strength, so you instinctually reach for the candy jar for the necessary energy to run.

Stress used to come from physical sources, like a hungry tiger charging your way. But today, you're more likely to be stressed by things that you can't fight or flee, such as unreasonable bosses or money troubles. So the sugar from candy just parks itself on your hips.

In addition, sugary foods increase serotonin, the feel-good neurotransmitter in the brain, so you feel calmer. "Sweet foods also release morphine-like substances that improve mood and reduce stress," says Amy Campbell, R.D., C.D.E., nutrition and diabetes educator at the Joslin Clinic at Harvard University.

Psychological theories say we eat sweets because they remind us of childhood times when we enjoyed them at a birthday party or Grandma's house. "It also has something to do with our primitive nature—a baby needs a nipple for food, and we need to stick something in our mouths to soothe ourselves," says Dr. Preuss.

**We need a lift.** "Many people use sweets as a pick-me-up when they're tired or doing something that requires concentration, like studying," says Dr. Dean.

Sugar also gives us a buzz. "There's a rise in beta-endorphins (chemicals that make us feel good) when we eat sugar," says Kathleen DesMaisons, Ph.D., president and CEO of Radiant Recovery in Albuquerque, and author of *The Sugar Addict's Total Recovery Program*. When the buzz wears off, cravings set in, she says.

And contrary to the popular belief that only depressed people eat for emotional reasons, happy people also down a few sweet treats to feel good. One study conducted at Case Western Reserve University showed that nondepressed university students ate cookies, as well as pretzels and cheese, because they thought the foods would boost their mood or help maintain an already good mood.

**Hormones take over.** Twenty-eight percent of women get food cravings compared with only 13 percent of men. Most men crave foods that combine fat and protein, like steak or Buffalo wings. But women yearn for sugary foods, like cheesecake and brownies, most likely because of female hormones.

For one, beta-endorphins drop right before a woman gets her period and during menopause, causing her to feel unhappy. "Eating sweets can be a pleasurable experience, and when you're feeling emotionally volatile, you may seek them," says Wright.

Also, women physically feel hungrier during PMS, and they get headaches, dizziness, and fatigue. So sugar may be a nice diversion from the *physical* discomfort.

**We're actually thirsty.** The urge for sugar could be masking a true need for water. "It's not uncommon for me to feel hungry for sugar only to find that the hunger promptly goes away when I drink a big glass of water," says Dr. Mabray. "Most of us tend to be flirting with dehydration as we try to find anything to drink *but* water."

**The more we get, the more we want.** Psychologically, the more you fight the cravings, the stronger they become. "The minute you tell people they can't eat a cookie or a piece of cake, that's all they want," says Campbell.

# Your Body Gets the Sugar Blues

Next time you sit down to a piece of cake, a bowl of ice cream, or a candy bar, pretend it's a martini and *then* decide whether or not to eat it. It's okay to have a glass or two of wine with dinner sometimes, but it's not okay to indulge all day, every day. The same goes for sweets.

Lots of sugar can take a toll on your health, leading to short-term problems like weight gain, increased appetite, and fatigue. Long term, too much sugar can promote nutrient deficiencies, obesity, diabetes, heart problems, tooth decay, and possibly even wrinkles. It takes roughly 10 to 20 years of steady consumption of refined sugar and junk food to put someone at risk for a chronic illness, says Carolyn Dean, M.D., N.D., a medical writer and media consultant in City Island, New York, and author of *Dr.*

*Carolyn Dean's Natural Prescriptions for Common Ailments.*

Although there is no scientific research to support their theroy, some alternative health practitioners believe that too much sugar causes yeast infections. Indeed, some of their patients believe that giving up sweets relieved their symptoms.

Some experts believe you should never add sugar to your oatmeal or enjoy a scoop of ice cream. But most nutritionists say that, in moderation, sugar is not an evil food. It just needs to know its place in your diet.

Here's how and why too much sugar leads to health problems, as well as how you can tell if your sugar consumption is putting you at risk.

## After Sugar Goes Down the Hatch

You probably don't think too much about a caramel sundae once your spoon hits the bottom of the dish. But your body has some work to do. Blood sugar rises, and your pancreas releases insulin. Like a stern principal, insulin grabs loitering sugar out of your bloodstream so it can't cause any trouble and pushes it into cells. (High blood sugar levels can cause health problems like heart disease and diabetes.) Cells use the sugar for energy, and blood sugar levels decrease again.

Thanks to this system, blood sugar usually stays under control. But if you eat too many sweets or are sugar sensitive, your blood sugar shoots up too high. Your body then produces too much insulin, your blood sugar drops too quickly, and you get tired, weak, and hungry.

It's hard to tell when you've overloaded on sugar because the brain is a sugar feeder. "You eat a doughnut and a Coke for breakfast, and your brain is flying high; but at the same time, sirens and whistles are going off in your body," says Rebecca Wright, R.D., L.D., at the Cancer Treatment Center of America in Tulsa, Oklahoma.

The brain and body battle. The brain says, "I like sugar . . . eat sugar!" But the rest of the body pleads with you to have some healthy fats, proteins, and vegetables.

## Crossing the "Too Much" Threshold

When asked how much sugar is too much, most dietitians and doctors say "tough question!" According to Wright, that's because some people are able to clear sugar out of their blood efficiently, while others cannot, because they're insulin resistant. In other words, their cells don't respond to insulin properly, so sugar stays in the bloodstream.

Here's how to recognize your sugar limits.

**Perform a test.** "Stop all added sugar and junk food for a week and then take a day (Saturday or another day when it won't interfere with work) and eat as much sugar as you want. See how you feel," says Dr. Dean. High blood sugar will likely manifest itself where you most often feel sick. "You may get a headache, clogged sinuses, or diarrhea," she says. But at least you'll know how the sugar affects you so you can tell when you've overloaded on it in the future.

**Calculate your intake.** The United States Department of Agriculture recommends limiting your sugar intake to between 6 and 10 percent of your total daily calories. That amounts to 6 teaspoons (24 grams) in a 1,600-calorie diet, 10 teaspoons (40 grams) in a 2,000-calorie diet, and 12 teaspoons (48 grams) in a 2,200-calorie diet.

Staying below your sugar "cap" may be tough, because so many foods are naturally or artificially sweetened. Consider that a single teaspoon of sugar equals 4 grams, a can of soda has 40 grams, and a serving of many cereals has 14 or more grams. If your breakfast consists of a bowl of cereal and a big mug of coffee with 2 teaspoons of sugar, you're close to your daily limit before you've even left the house.

The good news is that naturally occurring sugars—like fructose in fruits and vegetables and lactose in milk—do not count toward your 10 percent limit. Unfortunately, the labels on most foods lump naturally occurring sugars with added sugars when listing the total sugar content. To ferret out added sugars, check the ingredients list for names like high-fructose corn syrup, invert sugar, dextrose, barley malt, caramel, molasses, maltose, and honey.

**Take note of your fiber intake.** "Sugar is absorbed more slowly if it goes down with some fiber," says Harry Preuss, M.D., professor of physiology at Georgetown University School of Medicine in Washington, D.C. "In our studies, rats digest all the sugar when they eat it with fiber, but the sugar is less harmful because it's absorbed over a longer period of time rather than suddenly getting into the system." Shoot for at least 25 grams of fiber a day and try to eat fiber at the same time as sugar.

Keep in mind that eating too much sugar may overwhelm the benefits of fiber, Dr. Preuss adds. So if you eat 12 bags of candy, not even a whole box of All-Bran will slow it down.

**Examine the rest of your diet.** "The majority of your calories should come from foods packed with vitamins, minerals, protein, and carbohydrates," says Susan Kleiner, Ph.D., R.D., author of *Power Eating* and owner of High Performance Nutrition in Mercer Island, Washington. Then you can add some calories from sugar, she says.

**Monitor your movement.** The more calories you burn, the more you can eat. "If you work hard physically, sugar is great for maintaining energy in a fast, convenient way," says Therese Franzese, R.D., director of nutrition at the Peninsula Spa and Health Club in New York City. If you're out skiing all day, you can have a Gatorade or some candy because your body needs the extra calories. But if you spend most of the day (or week) motionless at your desk and in front of the TV, your body probably doesn't have room for empty sugar calories.

## Sugar's Short-Term Effects

Most of our added sugar is mixed in with our other food, so we can't always know for certain how it makes us feel. But symptoms like headaches, insomnia, and PMS can all be the result of too much sugar. "For example, I have a friend who's a total sugar addict. He says he's fine, but he has horrible allergies that, in my opinion, could very well be from the sweets," Dr. Dean says.

Here are some specific short-term effects of too much sugar.

**Fatigue.** When you eat a sweet, you feel great at first. "But once a lot of insulin is released, most of the sugar disappears, and you experience a drop in energy," says Dr. Dean. So you eat more sugar to get another boost. This sugar cycling throughout the day can make you feel very tired by evening.

Fatigue can also result from dehydration. "You use up a lot of water to process sugar metabolically," says Wright. So when your blood sugar is high, you become dehydrated.

Besides water, "you use up lots of B vitamins when you process sugar," adds Wright. B vitamins give you energy, so when you're deficient, you feel tired.

**Increased appetite.** Contrary to popular belief, candy bars don't satisfy your hunger for long. When blood sugar rises, resulting high insulin levels cause blood sugar to plummet. "Low blood sugar initiates hunger, light-headedness, and fatigue, prompting you to want more sugar or food," says Franca Alphin, R.D., clinical associate with the department of community and family medicine at Duke University in Durham, North Carolina.

In some people, artificial sweeteners seem to have a similar ef-

## ARTIFICIAL SWEETENERS: A GOOD ALTERNATIVE?

"Artificial sweeteners have not been around long enough for us to say it's definitely safe to drink 2 liters of diet soda a day," says Hillary Wright, R.D., nutrition coordinator for Harvard Vanguard Medical Associates in Boston. But like sugar, in moderation, artificially sweetened products are probably okay for most of us.

Some sugar substitutes, like aspartame (found in diet soda and sugar-free gum, yogurt, and pudding), are popular with dieters because they provide the sweet without the calories. But "sugar-free" doesn't *always* mean "calorie-free." For example, xylitol, an artificial sweetener used by people with diabetes because it requires little insulin to be metabolized, contains about half as many calories as sugar, with 2.4 calories per gram.

And most artificially sweetened foods don't offer much in the way of nutrition, so if you consume them, it's important to make sure that you're getting enough nutrient-dense foods. "A lot of the health problems we see these days have to do with what we're *not* eating—not just what we're getting too much of," says Wright.

Another thing to keep in mind is that artificial sweeteners can backfire in some people, making them hungrier for sugary sweets or other food. They can also cause diarrhea and cramping in some people. If you experience any of these side effects, try not to overdo it. Limit yourself to a serving or two of artificial sweeteners a day.

fect. In a 1999 Dutch study, 10 healthy men consumed a drink sweetened with sugar, a drink sweetened with the sugar substitute aspartame, or a drink high in fat. Their appetites were measured after each. The men were hungrier after they drank the sugar-sweetened and the aspartame-sweetened beverages than when they had the high-fat beverage.

**Weight gain.** Sugar itself doesn't cause weight gain. "I meet a lot of very thin people who eat a lot of sugar—it's just a calorie game," says Hillary Wright, R.D., nutrition coordinator for Harvard Vanguard Medical Associates in Boston. The problem is that sugary foods serve up a bunch of empty calories, and often we don't know when to stop. Many sweets, like soda and candy, don't satisfy our hunger. So our bodies don't hold back at dinner to make up for that afternoon soda and pack of Starburst.

Let's say you added a large soda to your diet every day and kept everything else the same. You'd gain over 3 pounds in less than a month.

"And a lot of sweets, like cookies, cake, and chocolate bars, are also high in fat, so you get even *more* calories," says Hillary Wright.

**Immune system suppression.** "Studies show that 20 teaspoons of sugar (the amount in two cans of soda) paralyzes 92 percent of your white blood cells for 5 hours," says Dr. Dean. Sugar doesn't kill the cells, but it puts them in a temporary trance, so viruses, bacteria, and other invaders can slip past them and make you sick.

## Long-Term Effects of a High-Sugar Diet

Things get worse, health-wise, if you've got a long-standing sugar habit. Here's what might head your way.

**Obesity.** It's easy to blame dietary fat for obesity—it serves up 9 calories per gram versus sugar's 4. But sweets shouldn't get off scot-free by any means. In fact, they seem to be *more* at fault for our expanding tummies than dietary fats, because many of us eat more sugar than fat. Thanks to the fat-free craze of the 1990s, we've replaced fat with far too much sugar. As a percentage, fat intake has declined since 1960, and sugar intake has sharply risen.

In a study done at the Harvard School of Public Health, 548 children between ages 11 and 17 were monitored for sugar-sweetened beverage intake and obesity for 1½ years. For every additional sugary drink they consumed, both their body mass index and obesity risk increased by 60 percent, regardless of their other dietary and lifestyle habits.

**Insulin resistance and type 2 diabetes.** "Some studies have shown that if you eat a lot of sugar for a number of years, you have a tendency to develop a resistance to insulin," says Dr. Preuss. Insulin resistance leads to elevated glucose and insulin levels in the blood, both of which are associated with type 2 diabetes, heart disease, high blood pressure, and periodontal disease.

Also, excessive sugar intake increases diabetes risk in people who are predisposed to the disease. Too much sugar often forces the pancreas to constantly release insulin to distribute the sugar load. One theory is that an overworked pancreas loses its ability to respond with the needed insulin, which leads to diabetes, says Dr. Dean.

And a high sugar intake can lead to obesity, another cause of diabetes. Fat tissue influences other tissues to become insulin resistant.

**High blood pressure.** "There's a link between high sugar intake and high blood pressure," says Dr. Preuss. In a study done at Georgetown University Medical Center, Dr. Preuss and his colleagues fed 225 rats one of five diets: a high-sugar, low-protein diet; a high-sugar, low-fat diet; a low-sugar, high-protein diet; a low-sugar, high-fat diet; and a diet containing moderate amounts of fat, protein, and sugar. The highest blood pressure readings were found in the rats that ate the two high-sugar diets.

**Heart disease.** In one large study, researchers spent 10 years tracking the health status of 75,521 women between the ages of 38 and 63, none of whom had previous diagnoses of heart attack, angina, stroke, diabetes, or other cardiovascular diseases. As part of the study, the researchers calculated the glycemic load for each woman, based on how often she ate sugar and other refined foods, as well as how much she ate of those foods.

Over the course of 10 years, 761 women developed coronary heart disease. Of these cases, 208 were fatal and 553 nonfatal. The researchers determined that a high glycemic load was directly associated with coronary heart disease.

**Magnesium deficiency.** Refined sugar weakens the pancreas by stimulating excessive insulin production. It also taxes the adrenal glands as they try to keep blood sugar balanced. In theory, at least, overworking these organs can lead to many deficiencies and imbalances, especially in the mineral magnesium. To make matters worse, the actual process of refining sugar from sugar cane or other natural sources removes most of the mineral content, including up to 99 percent of the magnesium.

**Other nutrient deficits.** Most sugary foods provide nothing nutritious. "You'll become nutrient-deficient if you continue to choose sweets over real, whole foods," says Franzese. Cells can survive and work well for only so long without the necessary nutrients—like copper, zinc, iron, and calcium (the list goes on and on)—before they start to break down. "There's nothing wrong with eating some chocolate every day. It's what you're doing the rest of the day that counts," notes Franzese.

**Tooth decay.** The dentist was right—sugar is bad for your teeth. When sugary foods hang out on your teeth after a meal or snack, bacteria form acids that eat away your tooth enamel. "I heard a dentist on the radio say that he sees more teenagers with cavities between their teeth than he's seen in 30 years of practice, and he thinks it's from drinking soda every day," says Dr. Kleiner.

**Wrinkly skin.** Sugar may even damage your skin by causing collagen, the protein that gives skin its elasticity, to become stiff and inflexible. This can lead to wrinkling.

Of course, none of this means you should never touch another éclair or piece of saltwater taffy again. We have a natural desire for sweets, and we shouldn't fight it. "People who continually deprive themselves get into a binge cycle," says Amy Campbell, R.D., C.D.E., nutrition and diabetes educator at the Joslin Clinic at Harvard University in Boston. If you want to eat some M&M's, go ahead. Just limit yourself to a few. Sweets are one of life's great indulgences. We can preserve them as special treats by giving them special places in our diets and our lives.

# Take Control of Your Sweet Tooth

# *SHE MADE A DATE*
# *TO GIVE UP SUGAR*

Jennifer Pruden can tell you the exact date she gave up sugar: February 23, 2001, just 1 month after her wedding anniversary and days shy of Lent. And just like the traditional carnival that preceded Lent in her native home of Panama, Jennifer made sure to binge on all her favorite sweets before quitting cold turkey on that magical day.

"It's like you party until it's time to give it up, and then you just give it up," says Jennifer, 26, of Meigs, Georgia.

Picking a day to quit helped Jennifer launch her new sugar-free life. Until then, she had led a sweet existence. She grew up surrounded by fields of sugarcane and turned into a chocoholic and Pepsi fiend as an adult. "I loved making desserts and eating them," she says. "I always had candy at my desk, peppermints and lollipops. And sometimes, I could eat a whole bag of Mint Milanos."

Shortly after she got married in 1997, Jennifer started gaining weight, putting on 50 pounds in 1 year. That led to a 3-year struggle with dieting. At one point, she was doing aerobics 5 days a week. But she didn't lose a pound, even after 7 months. It wasn't until doctors discovered she was insulin deficient that Jennifer realized she had a condition that impaired her body's ability to process sugar.

At that point, Jennifer read *Sugar Busters!* and decided to give the diet a try. She gave herself a week to clean out all sweets from her cabinets and desk drawers. "The week before, I just gorged myself," she says. "I even bought an extra bottle of wine, because I knew I had to give that up, too."

After unloading all her goodies, Jennifer turned to fruits, Triscuits, and V-8 juice in place of sweets. She traded her dinnertime glass of wine for a cup of green tea. And if she felt a sugar craving in the evening, she reached for plain instant oatmeal and hot tea. "That calms down any craving," she says.

A few weeks later, the cravings disappeared, Jennifer says. She slept better, felt more energetic, and no longer had mood swings or PMS. She also lowered her heart rate and her blood pressure. And after just 6 weeks, she shed 22 pounds, bringing her down to 217 on her 5-foot-6 frame.

Jennifer still wants to lose another 74 pounds, and she's confident she can do it. "I had made losing weight my New Year's resolution, and I was going to give up something for Lent anyway," she says. "By picking a date to give up sugar, I set a deadline for myself."

## WINNING ACTION

**Pick a day to give up sweets and mark it on your calendar.** *Setting a deadline or making an appointment with yourself will help you launch your effort to eliminate sugar from your diet. Spend the days leading up to it by going through your kitchen cabinets, refrigerator, and desk drawers, tossing out all sugary foods. After you've cleaned house, think of yourself as a new, sugar-free person.*

# SHE TOOK NOTE OF SUGAR'S EFFECTS

Most people carry grocery lists to the supermarket. Diane Bradshaw takes a list of all the bad things sugar does to her body. By reading it before she strolls past the cookies, ice cream, and

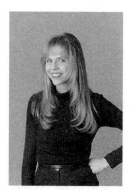

Diane has been sugar-free for 18 years.

brownies that were once a major part of her diet, Diane has been able to give up the sugar that once consumed her life.

Diane, who's 53 and lives in Salt Lake City, describes herself as a former sugar addict. "I was the type who said, 'Don't feed me dinner, feed me dessert,'" she says. "Oh sure, I ate my dinner, but my mind was focused on dessert."

Diane learned early on that sugar was not a good food. Her father was an orthodontist. She remembers him arriving home one day and tossing out all the sugar and white flour in the house. But he forgot to ditch the ice cream, which soon became Diane's biggest passion. "I ate at least a pint a day," she says. "I just didn't have the ability to stop."

At 15, Diane moved to New York City to train as a ballet dancer and became "totally hooked" on sugar. Dancing allowed her to devour sweets from Manhattan pastry shops and delis with reckless abandon. But when she stopped dancing, got married, and had her five children, sugar began to take its toll.

"After my first child arrived in 1971, I was sick with strep throat constantly, and I had colds and the flu all the time," she says. "I always felt like I needed more sleep, and I couldn't think clearly. It was a constant battle that left me feeling like I had no willpower and was out of control."

But bad health was not enough to keep Diane away from sweets, even as she began to suspect that sugar was contributing to her ailments. She felt as if she simply had no control over her addiction. "I noticed that when I went to the store and saw the ice cream, it was as if I went brain-dead and forgot why I shouldn't be eating it," she says. "So one day in 1981, I decided to write it all down."

On her list, she wrote that sugar sapped her energy, compromised her immune system, and obliterated her memory. She reminded herself that sugar left her in bed with bad colds and flu and muddied her ability to think clearly.

Whenever she was in the supermarket on the brink of buying ice cream, in a restaurant contemplating dessert, or at home about to plow through a bag of cookies, Diane would pull out her list and review her reasons for giving up sugar. The list conjured up images of Diane in bed with a nasty case of strep throat. "I'd pull out that list and say to myself, 'Is this what you want?'" she says.

It wasn't, and as sugar gradually lost its grip on Diane, her health improved. She noticed immediate changes—more energy, a better memory, and a decrease in the amount of time she spent sick in bed. After 2 months, she lost her cravings for sugar, and within a year, her memory of what it tastes like was gone. "Eventually, I didn't even care about it," she says. "Now, I haven't eaten any significant sugar in 18 years. I can look at desserts as if they are just objects."

### WINNING ACTION

**Write down the reasons you want to cut back on sugar.** *Carry the list with you at all times. Be brutally honest about how sugar makes you feel and what physical symptoms it provokes. Pay attention to whether you have more illness when you eat sugar than when you give it a wide berth. Whenever you feel the urge to* *buy or eat something sweet, pull out your list and re-mind yourself what you'll gain by saying no to the sweet stuff.*

## *SHE FOUND HER TRIGGERS AND SHOT DOWN HER SUGAR HABIT*

Kelly Kissane was faced with a frightening ultimatum in May 2000. "My eye doctor said I could either quit eating sugary foods or go blind," recalls the 39-year-old Ph.D. student from Reno, Nevada. "My eyes were starting to show signs of my diabetes, despite the fact that I am not insulin dependent."

A doctor first suspected that Kelly had type 2 diabetes when she was 20, but family problems prevented her from getting a full round of blood tests. Since a simple blood test indicated she was not dia-betic, she snacked for years without restraint. Pastries, candy, and ice cream became daily treats. But after learning that her eyes showed reversible symptoms of diabetes—leaky blood vessels causing a constant stream of floaters in her vision—she quit sweets cold turkey.

"It was hell for several months," admits Kelly. She faced count-less temptations from snack bars, vending machines, and well-meaning staff members. "The department secretaries always had a bowl of candy out for the graduate students," says Kelly, who used to dip into it three or four times a day.

As a biology student, she took a scientific approach toward tackling her incessant cravings: She sought to determine exactly what triggered them. "I am by nature insatiably curious. I often analyze myself, wanting to know how I tick. This was just another experiment," she says.

Her first observation? Just *seeing* candy fueled her desire to eat it. The quickest remedy? Steer clear of the departmental candy bowl. When she had to pass it, "I avoided looking at it," she says. She also shunned vending machines and the student union, where sweets abounded, choosing instead to brown-bag it or leave campus at mealtime. It worked. "If sweets are out of sight, the cravings don't overwhelm me," she says.

Her next observation: Both caffeine and aspartame-sweetened sodas brought back that snacking feeling. "I recognized the pattern and found alternatives like Hansen's natural sodas and SoBe lean drinks, which don't produce the same reaction," she says.

During an Internet search on diabetes, she discovered the glycemic index, which ranks foods according to how quickly they turn into blood sugar. Victuals that top the list and can stimulate sugar cravings include potatoes and white bread, both among Kelly's preferred foods at that time. She began using oat flour and other grains to prepare her own breads, rather than relying on store-bought loaves. She also added fiber-rich foods, such as strawberries, artichokes, and asparagus, to her daily menu. Those kept her feeling full "so I didn't feel the need to eat sugar or anything else," she says.

Kelly has maintained a largely sugar-free diet since July 2000, enabling her to successfully control her diabetes and reverse the blood vessel damage in her eyes. The floaters in her field of vision decreased in both number and size in just 8 months. "Now, I find even some diet drinks taste too sweet for me!" she insists.

*W I N N I N G   A C T I O N*

**Identify your triggers—then avoid them.** *Want to stomp out your appetite for sweets? Pay close attention to your body. When you find your mouth watering, ask yourself, "What brought this on?" Is it the mere sight of sweets? Does even one taste lead to an all-out binge? Does watching food commercials propel you off the sofa and into the kitchen? Once you have an answer, take steps to dodge situations and eliminate foods that spark cravings. Stay away from places where you have easy access to candies, cakes, and cookies. Channel surf away from the tempting ads—or better yet, get up during the break and walk around the house. To find out how your favorite foods rank on the glycemic index, check the Web or diet books.*

# SHE USES LABELS
# TO WEED OUT SUGAR TRAPS

Peggy Ward admits to being a longtime binge eater. "I could sit down with a whole bag of chocolate-covered peanuts and finish it off in 10 minutes," she says. "Or a Hershey bar with almonds, no problem."

Although she's been overweight much of her life, Peggy decided to do something about it in 1998, when she joined Weight Watchers. She stayed with it for 2 years and had some success in controlling her binges. "The program told us to eat what we wanted in moderation rather than gorging ourselves," says Peggy, who's 47 and lives in Tamarac, Florida. "I learned to tone down my gorging and feel satisfied with three little Tootsie Roll pieces for dessert. Compared with nothing, three was fabulous."

Stopping the binges was great progress, but Peggy soon discovered that was just the first step in cutting sugar out of her life. Her next step came after reading *Get the Sugar Out* by Ann Louise Gittleman, when she realized how many hidden sweeteners there are in most processed foods. "Now that I've made myself more aware, I read labels to see how much sugar is in each item," she says. A regular glass of milk, she points out, contains 12 grams of sugar. "Things like that just floored me," she says.

"The most interesting thing I found was that when an item is labeled low-fat, it usually contains more sugar than the 'regular' version," Peggy continues. "I was thinking that a food with little or no fat had to be better for me, until I saw how much sugar there was. Unbelievable!"

Peggy now spends a lot more time looking at nutrition labels to ensure that she doesn't eat anything that contains more than 2 or 3 grams of sugar per serving. She also does more shopping on the outside aisles of the supermarket—the produce, meat, and dairy sections—and avoids the pitfall of processed foods that make up the middle of the store. Milk, which was already a minor part of her diet, is out completely, and she's found an ice cream that contains only 3 grams of sugar.

Peggy has been reading labels and cutting out hidden sugars since 2000. "I feel so much better," she says. "I don't have these peaks where I'm real hyped up followed by deep lows, so that puts less of a strain on my body. I'm less tired because I'm on an even keel. I've lost about 10 pounds, too. I can feel the weight loss, as well as see it in the way my clothes fit.

"I am now totally in tune with my body," Peggy adds. "I just wish I had done this a lot earlier in my life. I would have been a lot healthier."

### WINNING ACTION

**Choose foods with no more than 3 grams of sugar.** *This isn't possible when you eat out, of course. But by paying more attention to nutrition labels in supermarkets, you'll become a better judge of which foods to avoid in all situations. The foods you choose might still contain plenty of carbohydrates, but as long as you aim low on the amount of sugar, you'll help reduce the highs and lows that your body goes through during a sugar-filled day.*

# SHE NOW EATS SWEETS WITHOUT SUBSTANCE

"Although I always knew I had poor eating habits, I was unwilling to make any changes because I really enjoyed sweets," says Lisa Vroman, of Barto, Pennsylvania. "I ate them most any time. I really loved the taste of chocolate!"

Lisa persisted in her dietary indiscretions until early 2001, when she was diagnosed with gestational diabetes while pregnant with her third child. At that point, she says, "I really didn't have a choice." She had to start eating more healthfully.

A mother with gestational diabetes can't produce enough insulin. The resulting increase in her blood sugar level stimulates insulin production in her fetus. The excess sugar that moves into the baby's cells can cause him to gain extra weight—and large babies often cause difficult and dangerous deliveries.

What's more, mothers who have had gestational diabetes are at greater risk for developing type 2 diabetes later in life. With that in mind, 37-year-old Lisa says, "You should try to keep to a sugar-free diet after giving birth. It should be a lifestyle change to avoid that risk."

To cut down on her sugar intake, Lisa stopped buying the peanut butter cookies and candy bars that she likes and instead bought only those sweets that the rest of her family enjoys. "I didn't want my family to sacrifice because I am unable to eat sweets," she says. "That really helped a lot."

But Lisa didn't want to cut sweet foods out of her diet completely. "After I was diagnosed, a nutritionist sat down with my husband and me to give us ideas of things we could eat that are still sweet," she says. The top treats that came out of that meeting were sugar-free Jell-O and pudding.

Although never a big Jell-O fan, Lisa gave the dessert a try and found that it really hit her sweet spot. "It was a 'free food,' one I could eat as much of as I wanted, and it's very sweet," she says, adding that it goes down even better with a dab of sugar-free whipped cream on top. "Sugar-free Jell-O and pudding have been real lifesavers for me because they allowed me to continue enjoying sweet treats."

Lisa's goal during her pregnancy was to keep her sugar intake to a minimum so she wouldn't have an oversized baby and difficult birth. This goal paid off on June 20, 2001, when her son was born, weighing in at 8 pounds 4½ ounces. But she resolved to continue her good habits after the delivery and has been successful so far. "I keep my sugar intake to a minimum and find I really don't crave sweets as much as I used to," she says.

*W I N N I N G   A C T I O N*

**Turn to sugar-free desserts.** *With no fat and low calories, sugarless Jell-O and puddings are guilt-free indulgences. They give you the sweetness you're craving and fill you up without packing on pounds. As replacements for typical desserts like cake and cookies, they're a satisfying way to shave heaps of sugar and loads of calories from your everyday diet. And you'll never suffer from going back for seconds! Keep an eye peeled when roaming the super-market aisles for other such foods. Remember to consult the Nutrition Facts label for sugar and calorie values and not rely on sensational claims on the front of the package.*

# SWEET DRINKS DON'T ENTICE HER ANYMORE

To some people, Sherry Granader might seem the picture-perfect image of health. She's been a nationally certified aerobics instructor for 17 years. She's written two books on healthy eating. And she hosts a radio show regularly to answer callers' questions about exercise and nutrition.

Sherry benefited from parents who kept her away from sodas when she was growing up. But as she got older, she found that she needed to pay still more attention to the sugar levels in her diet. "Around 1998, I noticed that keeping my body fat down was getting more difficult," says the 44-year-old Houston resident. "I was frustrated as to why that was happening, especially with all the classes I was teaching and my regular exercise."

After examining her diet more closely, Sherry decided she

needed to cut out the fruit juice she drank regularly. "I would have a glass of juice every day, but that's lots of sugar all at once—a couple hundred calories' worth. So I stopped that," she says. "After all, it's always better to eat the fruit instead of just drinking the juice. That significantly improved my physique. A 'cheat' for me became fresh-squeezed orange juice on Sundays."

In her role as a nutrition counselor, Sherry now encourages her clients to eat more fresh fruit—and not to overdo the juice. "A lot of them think it's healthy no matter how much they drink," she says. "But if they're not going to burn it off—which they're often not—then it's too high in sugar content."

### WINNING ACTION

**Limit the amount of sweets you sip.** *Anyone who's worrying about sugar consumption has probably already set aside regular soda for a diet version. (You've done this, right?) But plenty of commercial fruit drinks contain just as much sugar as soda—and you might be consuming too much of them since the word* fruit *may often imply health benefits. By eating the fruits themselves—oranges, apples, bananas, strawberries, and more—you get fiber and a host of nutrients. And if you're still thirsty after your snack, turn to water instead of something sweet to rinse your palate. Your body will thank you.*

## SHE'S GONE SOUR ON SUGAR

Jill Quick had been waging a war against weight gain for more than three decades. But no matter how she struggled, the weight

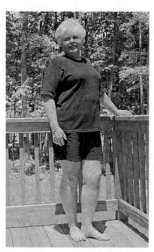

Since giving up sugar, Jill can fend off colds better.

kept winning. "Since my pregnancies, I have dieted, starved, exercised, and read many books trying to understand why I couldn't eat normal quantities of food without gaining rapidly," she says. "At age 34, I was about 70 pounds above my desired weight."

The key to Jill's weight problem lay in that phrase "since my pregnancies," but no one recognized that until long after the damage had been done. "I would be berated for gaining weight when I went for checkups and had no help with trying to understand what was going wrong with my metabolism," she says. "Needless to say, this made me very upset."

In 1998, Jill's doctor determined that she probably developed gestational diabetes during her pregnancies, which has caused her weight problems. That discovery brought with it a solution to her woes: Cut out sugar completely. "I was trying to have small balanced meals, but they never worked for me," she says. "Even though I don't have diabetes, I've been told that my body can't handle a lot of carbohydrates. I have to go as low carb as possible to make my metabolism work."

Jill says that sugar cravings are a thing of the past now. "There are many tricks to fool the palate and change your cravings," she says. "I have found the best one for me is to eat a dill pickle. The sour taste kills my craving for a sweet.

"Drinking a full glass of water with lemon in it helps also," Jill continues. "Citrus seems to cut the sweet attack. I don't feel it is helpful to substitute other sweet tastes. As long as you have weight to lose, it is better to eliminate the need for a sweet taste."

Since deep-sixing sugar (and almost all refined carbs) from her diet, this 58-year-old resident of Midlothian, Virginia, has lost 30 pounds, bringing her down to 186 on her 5-foot-6 frame. "I have 36 pounds to go," Jill says. "My doctor is thrilled that I've gotten any weight off with my unusual metabolism."

And her immune system is much stronger now. "I can fight off colds and sickness within a few days, about half the normal expected rate," Jill says.

*WINNING ACTION*

**Grab something sour to kill the craving.** *Trying to fool your sweet tooth with a substitute for what you're craving might not work for you and might leave you unsatisfied. If that's the case, overwhelm the desire with a strong appeal to your other taste buds. Sour foods generally have fewer calories than sweet ones. And you have to admit that you're not nearly as likely to reach for a brownie after eating a dill pickle!*

# SHE PREFERS PRODUCE TO PASTERIES

Barbra Dickson had a passion for pastries, and in her old job at Albertson's supermarket, her plate never ran empty. "I knew the bakery manager there because I worked in the meat department," she says. She would take samples of cooked items over to him, and in exchange, he would set her up with scones, filled croissants, chocolate chip cookies—pastries of every shape and size.

When Barbra, who lives in San Angelo, Texas, took the job in early 2000, she thought she'd lose weight from moving around all day. But as she says, "That was definitely not the case." By February 2001, she had left Albertson's, moving away from the constant temptation of the pastries and into a healthier way of eating.

"I had always been basically a vegetarian," says Barbra, but the discovery of a cassette tape touting the benefits of raw foods gave this 29-year-old a new diet model to work with. "Usually, people don't equate raw foods with an actual recipe except a salad," she explains. "But I found a whole cuisine out there"—one rich in recipes that explain how to incorporate nuts, herbs, and seeds into a diet in creative ways. It's nothing like eating the same salad every single day.

"For the first week or so when you start eating vegetables, your body may want to go back to what it was doing. But if you keep at it, your desire for different types of food will change," says Barbra. Whereas she used to get hit with cravings for something sweet, now her desires range to more specific foods, like apples or cucumbers. "You crave a bigger variety of things. You can tell in your body that you don't need 'just sugar' anymore."

Now that approximately half her diet is raw fruits and vegetables, Barbra says she's noticed some important changes in her body. "One thing is that I don't eat as much," she says. "If I eat a salad or one of my nut pâtés, it seems to fill me up a lot faster than when I cooked everything."

Barbra says that the raw foods also help her avoid that "heavy" feeling in her stomach that often accompanied cooked food. "That's a feeling most people get used to, but it isn't healthy," she says. "My meals are lighter and easier to digest."

What's more, Barbra no longer grabs pastries for quick energy. "As a matter of course now, I'm eating a lot of stuff that provides a more steady source of energy," she says. "It's more of an even keel."

### WINNING ACTION

**Eat veggies with abandon.** *This doesn't mean limiting your diet to carrot sticks and celery. Numerous cookbooks abound that demonstrate how to use nuts, herbs, and spices to make satisfying meals based on greens and other vegetables. These foods contain nearly no sugar, natural or otherwise, so they don't adversely affect your blood sugar. And a garden-based meal will also help you feel full longer—so you're less likely to reach for sweets between meals.*

# A DIET DIARY HELPS HER STAY ON TRACK

Rosie O'Neill had been thin for all of her 21 years—but that didn't stop her from changing her diet for the better.

"In early 2000, I noticed that I had become incredibly dependent on sugar as a source of energy," says Rosie, who lives in Los Angeles. "I didn't eat large quantities of candy or sugar at a time, but I snacked on little handfuls of candy throughout the day. If I hadn't had any in a couple of hours, my energy level would sink very rapidly!"

Rosie also noticed that she was having a harder time staying in shape, even though she exercised often. "I wanted to get the full potential out of my workouts and my otherwise healthy diet," she says.

To help her get away from snacking, Rosie put her college education to work. For a nutrition and physiology class she took at UCLA, she had to develop and analyze her own nutritional profile. "We were instructed to write down everything we ate for a week," she says. The exercise convinced Rosie that she needed to cut back on sugar.

"I bought a bunch of little notepads and started writing everything down," Rosie recalls. "If I walked to the snack cabinet at work and grabbed a handful of M&M's, I wrote that down. If I took a couple of Gummi Bears out of the jar on my boss's desk, I wrote that down. Writing down every single thing I ate really forced me to identify exactly how much candy I had over the course of a day—and it was a lot!"

In fact, after calculating everything she ate on her first day of diary dieting, Rosie realized she had eaten the equivalent of more than five candy bars. "It was ridiculous!" she says.

"Writing things down forced me to think twice when my hand was reaching for the candy jar," she adds. "If I was about to grab a handful of Mike and Ike candy, my first thought would be, 'Okay, I'm going to have to write this down. Do I really need this candy? Do I even want it?' Usually, the answer was no."

In addition to making Rosie think more about her cravings, the journal also provided a record of the progress she made. "When I'd see my sugar intake decreasing in my journal, it gave me a feeling of accomplishment, like I had really taken charge of something and fixed it."

Rosie no longer documents her diet now that she has developed the self-discipline to resist sugar cravings. While her weight was not a motivator to give up her sugar-chomping ways—she was already thin—her body has changed nevertheless. "I feel much more toned, my body feels lighter, and my clothes fit better," she says. "Overall, I just feel more healthy."

## W I N N I N G   A C T I O N

***Write down everything that you eat.*** *Everything! Count the number of M&M's, measure the volume of the brownies, stack the empty soda cans on the kitchen counter. By recording the extent of your sweet tooth in every way possible, you become more accountable for your diet and your overall health. The effervescence of the sugar may evaporate quickly, but the permanence of your honeyed history will leave a trail you won't be able to forget so easily.*

# HER MENTAL IMAGE OF SUGAR KEEPS SWEETS AWAY

Christy Havranek studied animation in college. So when she decided to cut sugar from her diet, she used a bit of mental animation, creating an image of what sugar was doing to her body. "I could see things moving that usually aren't moving," she says.

Christy, who's 23 and lives in Brooklyn, was a 17-year-old high school junior when she learned she had fibromyalgia, a condition that causes fatigue, muscle pain, and stiffness. Once diagnosed, she scoured the Internet and pored over literature from her health-care providers, quickly educating herself about the effects of nutrition on her health. Her research and experience led her to believe that excess carbohydrates might worsen her condition. She had already noticed that sugar, like other carbohydrates, made her sluggish and tired.

Armed with this theory, Christy gradually removed sugar from her diet. "I started by cutting out regular sweets," she says. "Then I progressed to getting rid of all refined sugar, which I'm still working on."

Although Christy never ate enormous amounts of sugar, she did enjoy her share of candy and cookies. And she had gotten away from them for months at a time in the past. "I've always had a sweet tooth," she says. "So it's been really hard to pull myself away from excess sugar and sweets permanently."

These days, Christy battles sugar cravings almost every day. She works in an office where everyone is wild about sweets and brings in treats to share. So when temptation strikes, Christy munches on an apple instead. If she's home, she plays music, sings, or paints to distract herself.

When her cravings get really bad, she creates a mental image of sugar in her body. "I think of it as something really viscous going through my veins," she says. "I think of it slowing me down."

Since cutting back on sweets, Christy has lost 20 pounds. At 5 feet 3 inches tall, she weighs about 160—and most of that is lean muscle, built by working out for an hour a day three or four times a week.

While Christy is eating less sugar than she used to, she hasn't gone cold turkey. Occasionally, especially during a bad bout of PMS, she allows herself to enjoy a sweet—only to get a headache that strengthens her resolve to stay sugar-free.

# *SHE COOKED UP A PLAN TO CUT BACK ON SUGAR*

Some people consciously reduce the sugar in their diets. Ginny McEwen let it slowly diminish. Once she started cooking and realized how much sugar went into a pie or cookie recipe, she could easily make more nutritious choices.

"Sometimes, I couldn't even get past reading the recipe," says Ginny, 59, of Albany, New York. "I thought, 'This just can't be.'"

As a child, Ginny had a penchant for her father's homemade fudge, and she loved eating hot-fudge sundaes. But as a young adult in the 1960s, she—along with her husband—became a vegetarian. Her husband was on a sentient yoga diet, which required Ginny to cook everything from scratch and prohibited any processed, packaged foods. To save money, they joined the Cambridge Food Conspiracy, a Massachusetts-based food co-op, and bought fruits and vegetables in bulk.

Back then, Ginny knew little about cooking but immediately realized that she liked it. So she started taking cooking classes, learned more about food and nutrition, and traded recipes with friends. Ginny gave baking a try but quickly discovered that most recipes required two-thirds to a whole cup of sugar. She knew from her research that sugar was nothing but empty calories. "There was just such a guilty feeling about that much sugar," she says.

Doing her own cooking also led her to cut down on snacking. Ginny had neither the money nor the interest in buying sweets. "When you shop with the intent of cooking your own food, you tend to buy whole ingredients," she says. "You just don't keep boxed cookies and crackers in the house. If you want something like that, you have to make it."

Soon, eating any kind of sugar resulted in a stomachache or headache, and sweets simply disappeared from her meals. Although it's been about 30 years since sugar first started fading from her life, Ginny still gets occasional cravings, which she usually attributes to fatigue or nerves. "It's usually a clue that something's not right, and I just need to sit down, rest, and relax," she says.

Desserts are a rare treat in the McEwen home. Instead, Ginny will cut up a mango to share with her husband or dig into a big salad with a new kind of dressing. In the summer, she occasionally indulges in ice cream but is more likely to munch on fruits. When she does bake, she prefers oatmeal raisin cookies or cookies made with sweet potatoes and honey. The one time she still bakes with sugar is in the spring, when Ginny makes her rhubarb pie. "Other sweeteners just didn't work," she says.

# SHE BEATS SUGAR BY THE BOOK

When Theresa Pancerz was diagnosed with type 2 diabetes in January 2000, at age 72, she made up her mind then and there to change her ways. "I'm not ready to die of diabetes," she says.

Theresa's blood sugar levels had been a bit high for years, "especially during the holidays," she says. "I'd eat a little bit of candy here and a few more cookies there."

But once the LaCrosse, Wisconsin, resident was diagnosed with diabetes, she cut out most of the sweets and began using a diabetic cookbook for meal ideas. Surprisingly, she says, the preparation and taste of the food weren't all that different from what she had been accustomed to. "I do miss the candy and cookies now and then," Theresa admits. "But the diabetic cookbook has recipes for cookies and other sweet things specifically for people with diabetes, so actually, I'm not missing too much."

Two treats that Theresa especially enjoys are Jell-O and milk shakes. "I use fat-free milk, fruit, ice cubes, and a little Sweet'N Low.

It makes a wonderful shake," she says. "I can fill up on that without gaining weight, and the sugar count stays down."

As for the Jell-O, Theresa has a unique way of preparing it. "I use the sugar-free kind and add lots of vegetables, like celery, radishes, carrots, and cabbage," she says. "I remember seeing it in restaurants a long time ago but was never apt to eat it then. Now, I get my dessert and veggies at the same time, and it takes care of that little craving I get."

Within a year of starting her new diet, Theresa—who's 5 feet 3 inches—lost 36 pounds, bringing her down to 175. More important, the weight loss and low-sugar diet helped stabilize her blood sugar levels.

"For people who have been eating sweets all their lives, giving up sugar is hard," says Theresa. "But I know I'm doing something right for me, and that makes me feel good all over."

### WINNING ACTION

***Turn to diabetic cookbooks for low-sugar meals.*** *Even if you've never worried about your blood sugar level, take a cue from those who know best how to monitor their sugar intake. Most diabetics don't forgo sugar completely, so there will still be plenty of sweet treats in the cookbooks—but those treats will be better for you because they'll have less sugar. If nothing else, you can compare recipes in diabetic cookbooks with those in regular cookbooks and learn how to reduce the amount of sugar you use in every meal you make.*

# *TO AVOID SUGAR, SHE EATS LIKE CLOCKWORK*

In 1998, while still in graduate school, Cid Szegedy took on modeling assignments to help out with her tuition. The work boosted her bank account, but her health paid the price as she strived to maintain her 5-foot-8-inch, size-2 body.

"I stopped eating to stay thin and achieve a sense of control, and as a result, I became very ill," she says. "I would go for 5 days without eating, but at the same time, I was addicted to exercise.

"Naturally, when you starve your body, you experience wild cravings because you're not getting any calories," Cid adds. And what she craved was cookies—specifically, chocolate chip cookies. "It was like a high because I would eat massive amounts of sugar and starch for a couple of hours and then abstain again," Cid recalls. "My blood sugar was all over the place."

Finally, in the fall of 1998, after becoming light-headed and blacking out several times, Cid realized what she was doing to her body. With help from a nutritionist, she slowly eased into a balanced diet not loaded with sugar. "It was difficult because I put on weight—albeit healthy weight—and retained water," she says. "Even adjusting to a larger wardrobe was tough."

On her own, Cid started reading a lot about nutrition. She discovered how to eat normally without developing the wild cravings that plagued her in the past. "I now manage my diet, like everything else in my life. I eat small meals, anywhere from 200 to 400 calories, every 2 to 3 hours," she says. "There's some kind of security in knowing that every few hours I can have a little something."

In the morning, Cid typically drinks a protein shake. Small meals throughout the day often take the form of protein bars that contain at most 2 grams of sugar. "These bars are incredible, provided you read the label," she says. "Make sure that they don't have sugar because some of them are no better than candy bars." Dinner is usually a healthy piece of fish, such as salmon or tuna steak, and steamed vegetables.

Her new diet also calls for her to avoid "whites"—her term for pasta, flour, starch, and any bread that's not whole grain. "If I'm desperate, I'll opt for a nibble of whole-grain bread, but generally, I'll avoid it because it triggers something in my head and brain that makes me want more, more, more," she says.

Cid, now 27 and working as a public relations consultant in Washington, D.C., may be eating more than she used to, but that's not a concern for her anymore. "It's very important to feed your body every couple of hours because you need to keep the furnace fired. It's important to keep your metabolism going," she says. "If anything, I'm much healthier because I lost the water weight I gained with the initial changes in my diet and gained muscle from lifting weights on a regular basis."

### WINNING ACTION

**Plan on small meals throughout the day.** *If you spread your eating over all your waking hours, you're never far away from your next scheduled meal—which may make it easier to hold off on snacking. Small meals, especially ones high in lean protein, help you feel full longer and reduce your desire to head to the vending machine. Since you want to avoid spending all day in the kitchen, you'll probably need to eat prepared foods some of the time. If so, make sure to choose ones low in sugar for the best results.*

# A HEALTHY BREAKFAST HELPED HER DODGE MORNING SWEETS

Jenna Spear-O'Mara used to eat sugar every morning—a doughnut from Starbucks, pastries at a meeting, pancakes at a restaurant. These days, by filling up on a healthy breakfast at home, Jenna resists the temptation to pick up sweets as she makes her way through the A.M. hours.

Jenna, 30, of Keene, New Hampshire, has always loved sugar, especially anything made with chocolate. "I would get a candy bar every day, and I had a sugary treat at the end of every meal," she says.

In the early 1990s, Jenna started feeling light-headed on a daily basis. Sometimes, the feeling was so bad that she could barely drive. "It really affected my life, to the point where I felt disabled," she says. Doctors diagnosed her with neurocardiogenic orthostatic hypotension, a condition in which standing up causes a sudden drop in blood pressure, leading to dizziness, light-headedness, and blurred vision. Jenna began taking medications to control her symptoms.

By 1999, Jenna and her husband were ready to start a family, and she decided to see a nutritionist in the hopes of giving up the drugs. The nutritionist suggested she cut out all white flour and refined sugar. The next time Jenna caved in to a sugar craving and ate a bowl of chocolate ice cream, she paid dearly. "I was light-headed for a week," she says. "My cardiologist said I was extra sensitive to sugar."

Jenna became a voracious label reader and discovered refined sugar in foods she never suspected, even pasta sauce, creamed corn, and crackers. Whenever possible, she replaced these foods with sugar-free alternatives. She found she could satisfy her sweet tooth with treats like dried fruit, chocolates sweetened with rice syrup, and soy ice cream.

But to really cut out refined sugar, Jenna knew she had to change the way she ate in the mornings. Instead of picking up a doughnut with her cup of coffee at Starbucks, she sought out bagel shops. Rather than indulge in the pastries served at breakfast meetings, she carried fruit, especially apples or bananas, or yogurt for her own midmorning snack.

Most important, she loaded up on a healthy breakfast before leaving the house. These days, she typically eats a low-sugar, high-fiber cereal such as Grape-Nuts with milk, a sugar-free bran muffin sweetened with maple syrup, or some plain yogurt and fruit. If she happens to be eating out, she orders eggs, toast, potatoes, and fruit.

Bad memories of how sugar makes her feel help Jenna steer clear of sweets. "I know if I eat sugar I'll feel horrible," says Jenna, who did become pregnant after she quit the drugs and changed her diet. "But even if it didn't make me light-headed, I wouldn't go back. I feel so much better now and healthier."

## W I N N I N G   A C T I O N

**Make breakfast mandatory.** *Many people try to save time by forgoing their morning meal, but they may be short-changing themselves in the long run. They're vulnerable to dips in their energy levels and mood—and as a result, they're likely to reach for something sweet to tide them over until lunchtime. They may get an energy boost, but they're taking in lots of empty calories, too. A better bet is to eat a good breakfast, even if it means getting up a bit earlier in the morning. Just be wary of sugar-laden convenience foods like doughnuts, muffins, and toaster pastries, which can set the stage for midmorning cravings.*

# HE TRACKED HIS
# REACTIONS TO SUGAR

Bill Norwood keeps a health log. In it he records everything he eats, along with physical and mental symptoms he experiences during the day.

"I'm a scientific type of person, so I like to study and monitor myself in this way," says Bill, 60, a technician in the physics department at the University of Maryland at College Park. "I want to make a mental connection between what I eat and how I feel. It helps me understand my health better."

As a direct outcome of keeping his log, Bill was able to identify 17 specific changes in his body after he stopped eating sugar in January 1990. Among them: Cold and flu incidence was down 75 percent. Headaches, "almost a constant problem" before, were nearly gone, as were sinus problems, earaches, and sore throats.

He no longer needed the asthma shots that he had been getting regularly for 6 years. Cold sores and warts were things of the past; his trips to the dentist were more pleasant because there was less plaque buildup; and stomachaches, which he had suffered regularly, were gone. And these were not fleeting changes. Eleven years after Bill ate his last cookie, all 17 improvements were for the most part intact, he says.

"I believe my health problems were definitely related to sugar," he says. "I love ballroom dancing and swimming, but I couldn't do either because I would get short-winded. All that changed with no sugar."

Bill was always aware of the effects of food on health. As a young parent, he did not allow sweets in the house. But at work, where "vending machines were all over the place," and where the physics department sponsored daily afternoon teas, it was a different story. "I was invited to eat all the cookies I wanted at the tea, and I ate all the cookies I wanted," he says. "I tried to control it, I tried to eat less, but I just plain enjoyed it."

The turning point came after a sugar binge that left him nauseated. "I got angry because I had once again failed to control my sugar intake," he says. "That's when I decided I had to treat my sugar consumption as an addiction. Once I made that decision, I gave up sweets completely."

Bill lost 10 pounds in the months after he stopped eating sugar and other sweeteners. At 5 feet 11½ inches, he went from 165 pounds to 155. Since then, with a diet made up largely of salads, vegetables, fresh fruits, beans, grains, and fish, he has lost an additional 10 pounds.

"There is no question in my mind that this diet could benefit everyone," he says. "It was a big lift; I felt better than I had for 10 years. To be turning 50 and feel younger and have those headaches that were a constant for all those years be gone. . . it's nothing short of wonderful."

Bill says that he is no longer tempted to eat sugary foods. But if he is, all he need do is take a look at his log and review the symptoms that have disappeared since he stopped eating sugar.

"I feel better," he says. "And I know why."

## WINNING ACTION

**Be aware of the connection between what you eat and how you feel.** *The pleasure of eating a candy bar or a few cookies at an afternoon tea spans mere minutes. But the aftereffects are long-lasting. Being aware of those effects can help in the effort to resist those few minutes of pleasure. A health log is one way to accomplish that.*

*Seeing in black and white—or, with the help of a com-*
*puter, in bright colors and graphs—that headaches or*
*lethargy regularly hits soon after a sugar binge could be*
*a life-changing lesson.*

## SHE TUNED IN TO HERSELF— AND TUNED OUT ON SWEETS

Donna Rubinstein didn't set out to give up sugar. In fact, the 37-year-old freelance magazine editor and yoga instructor was never much of a sugar fiend to begin with. But meditating for just minutes a day put her in touch with her body's nutritional needs, and she gradually learned that she didn't need—or want—any sugar in her life.

"Once I cleansed my system, two or three cookies could make me feel jumpy," she says. "I haven't craved sweets since."

That wasn't always the case. Although Donna rarely ate sweets as a child, she did discover them in high school and college. "When I started living on my own, I used to have sundaes, cookies, and cakes," she says.

That began to change around 1995, when Donna took up reflexology. She followed it a year later with yoga. Every morning, as part of her yoga training, she sat cross-legged on the floor of her Manhattan apartment, closed her eyes, and tried to focus on her breathing. It wasn't easy at first, and Donna found her mind darting from her job to her boyfriend, even to what she was going to eat at lunch. But with daily practice, she learned to calm her restless mind and built up her meditation time to 20 minutes.

"Meditation and yoga helped me really get in touch with my-

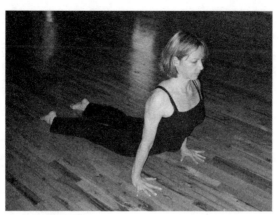

Donna credits yoga with curbing her appetite for sweets.

self," Donna says. "Once you understand who you are, you come to know why you behave the way you do, why you eat what you eat, and how that affects the way you feel."

Although she never intended to eliminate sugar from her diet, Donna did eventually give up all processed foods, devoting herself instead to eating fruits, vegetables, and grains. "I basically eat only things that grow from the ground or fall from a tree," she says.

Sugar no longer fits into that eating plan. Donna still keeps sweets in her kitchen for her boyfriend—she just has no desire to eat them. Instead, she munches on nuts, raisins, and granola. By cutting back on sugar, Donna realized she no longer even wanted sweets, especially since she felt more energetic. "Every time I ate sugar at a birthday party or on a special occasion, I felt bad," she says. "It made me really anxious and jumpy."

Even on her busiest days, Donna continues to devote time to meditating every morning. Meditation, she says, makes her aware that everything she does has an effect on her health.

## SHE FOUND A NEW PLAN TO KEEP SUGAR AT BAY

Tamarah Terral used to suffer regularly from hypoglycemia, or low blood sugar. "I was crashing every hour and a half," says the 29-year-old Warrenton, Virginia, resident. "I felt like I was falling apart—migraines, nausea, shakes, passing out, total exhaustion at all times."

In early 1999, her fiancé gave her a book on the Atkins diet, thinking it might address her troubles. "I skeptically took the book," Tamarah says—but once she read it, she thought she had nothing to lose by trying the program.

"The book said to reduce my intake of refined carbohydrates, white sugar, and starch," she recalls—and that proved to be a big change for her. "Before I changed my habits, I drank a 12-pack or more of regular Coca-Cola *daily*. Lots of bread and potatoes in some form daily. I often had juice and baked goods of varying kinds.

"Within 24 hours of cutting out these foods, all of my previously debilitating symptoms totally disappeared," Tamarah continues. "I was shocked. So that began a new life for me with radically reduced amounts of sugar and starch."

Currently, Tamarah works to maintain a diet that supplies fewer than 85 grams of carbohydrates per day. "To lose weight, I have to eat 60 or fewer grams of carbs per day," she says. "To just control my blood sugar, less than 85 grams per day does away with crashes and symptoms of any kind."

This means eating few potatoes and little corn, as well as avoiding white bread and regular pasta in favor of small amounts of the whole-grain, low-carb varieties. "I focus the majority of my eating on protein-rich meats and colorful vegetables high in vitamins and minerals—lots of greens, reds, and oranges," Tamarah says. She's also replaced the sugary soda with its diet twin and lots of water.

Now, when sugar cravings hit, Tamarah has new treats to reach for, ones that fit with her plan. "I make use of low-carb candy bars or European chocolate, which has a much lower sugar content than American chocolate," she says. "For dessert, I sometimes have soft French dessert cheeses, such as brie, which are sweet but not sugary. I also use Carnation fat-free hot chocolate mix, which is very low in sugar, to make different desserts, including cheesecake, parfaits, and hot chocolate."

These changes, in combination with the Atkins diet, helped Tamarah—who is 5 feet 8½ inches tall—lose 40 pounds in 1 year. After suffering for more than two decades, she can't get over how great she feels. "I cannot believe the difference in my life with such a small change," she says. "Missed family occasions and ruined vacations are now history thanks to a reduction in sugar. I am ecstatic. It has given me my life back."

### WINNING ACTION

**See if a lower-carbohydrate diet can help.** *If you suspect that carbohydrates may be triggering your sugar cravings, you may need to do more than cut back on high-sugar foods. Limit your intake of other carbohydrates like breads, pasta, cereal, and starchy vegetables. In their place, eat more lean protein so that you stay full longer. And have plenty of nonstarchy vegetables, like peppers, onions, greens, and such. Be careful about upping your intake of cholesterol and fat—you don't want to exchange one diet woe for another. In fact, check with your doctor, who may want to monitor you while you're cutting carbs.*

## *A LOW-SUGAR BREAKFAST STARTS HER DAY RIGHT*

For Jennifer Bright, just one change in her diet first thing in the morning set a healthy tone for the rest of her day. "I noticed that I was really tired and hungry all the time," she says. "I did some reading and put together the hunger, the fatigue, and the 15 pounds I'd put on—it was all due to my horrible diet."

That "horribleness" started first thing in the morning. "I eat the same thing every morning, for simplicity's sake. I just grab it and go," says Jennifer, who lives in Emmaus, Pennsylvania. Unfortunately, that simple breakfast was a pair of Tastykake chocolate cream-filled cupcakes—230 calories and most of it sugar. "It's probably the equivalent of eating 6 teaspoons of sugar in the morning—with a cup of coffee, no less," Jennifer notes ruefully.

"I discovered that the one quick and easy change I could make was to stop eating these cupcakes for breakfast every day," she continues. "So I started toasting a frozen waffle and putting peanut butter on top. I found that the combination of getting rid of a lot of sugar and having some protein from the peanut butter not only gives me more energy throughout the morning but also makes me more satisfied. I'm not starving by 10 A.M. as I was when I had a high-sugar breakfast."

And even when Jennifer does snack at 10:00, she now picks up a healthier item like an apple or other piece of fruit. "I find that if I eat sugar for breakfast, I'm craving something else sugary for my midmorning snack," she says. "So now I start the day off in a healthy way, which carries through for the whole day."

This 30-year-old has recently weaned herself from the frozen yogurt machine at work. Now when she craves a snack in the evening, she eats low-calorie popcorn after dinner instead of the cookies and cupcakes she used to nosh on.

"This is without question my best strategy," says Jennifer. "I crave sugar and sweets less throughout the day, and my energy's better."

### W I N N I N G   A C T I O N

**Start your day nutritiously.** *A breakfast of cupcakes, doughnuts, or sweetened cereal is one that's going to race through your system in no time flat since it's mostly sugar unaccompanied by protein or fiber. When you start the day with sweets, you'll undoubtedly find yourself ravenous by midmorning—which all too often translates into more sugar and an early lunch. But if your breakfast in-*

*cludes a source of lean protein and healthy fat like peanut butter or a hard-boiled egg, or if it's full of fiber as in a bran-type cereal, you'll keep your blood sugar level on an even keel and find yourself satisfied until lunch.*

# SHE CHEWED IT OVER AND CAME UP WITH THE SOLUTION

Nutritionist Allyson Mechaber has advice for people who are trying to eat less sugar. And it is the same advice mothers have been handing out for generations.

"I tell my clients to chew their food really well," says Allyson, who has a bachelor's degree in nutrition from Montclair State University in New Jersey and a master's in nutrition from New York University. "The more they chew, the sweeter and more flavorful starchy foods become."

This is especially true for carbohydrates like whole grains—brown rice in particular—and carrots and other vegetables. In those foods, starch changes to sugar with more mastication. "I tell people they should pay attention to what's happening as they keep chewing," Allyson explains. "Carbs taste sweeter, which makes them more satisfying."

It is not just through her schooling or helping people with sugar addiction that Allyson, 30, learned about the powers of thorough chewing. As a teenager, she ate a lot of sugar and refined foods. "I started my morning with a bowl of cereal, but I didn't realize it was loaded with sugar and stripped of nutrients," she says. "I also craved sweets and other processed foods all day. I was a big cookie eater."

While in her early twenties, Allyson experienced frequent bouts of nausea and fatigue. Eventually, she was diagnosed with irritable bowel syndrome and low blood sugar. "That's when I learned how to change my diet to one that was well-balanced and closer to nature," she says.

But it wasn't a simple process. "It was a constant battle," says Allyson, of Hasbrouck Heights, New Jersey. "It was something I had to work on for years. I was addicted to sugar, so if I had even a little bit, I got cravings all over again."

Allyson boosted her intake of low-fat proteins and started eating more unrefined carbs, especially vegetables and salads, which create a feeling of satiety.

Within a week of finally eliminating sugar from her diet, Allyson started feeling better. These days, she might have a sweet treat once a week. Even then, the misery that sometimes follows reminds her why she stopped eating sugar in the first place.

"It is so wonderful to feel well instead of unhealthy, to be energized and in a better mood," she says. "I crave sugar only occasionally now, because I eat right." And because those good-for-her foods get a good chewing, she adds.

"Everyone loves sugar," she says. "But too much wreaks havoc on our bodies. We are so used to feeling unwell that we don't even recognize it anymore. But once you beat a sugar addiction, you'll discover that you control how you feel, both physically and mentally."

## WINNING ACTION

**Thoroughly chew your foods.** *The longer you chew starchy foods, the sweeter they become and the more they satisfy your sweet tooth. Chewing is the first step in* *the digestive process. During chewing, an enzyme changes some of the starches in the food to sugar, producing the sweet flavor. Chewing has other benefits as well, including easing the workload of organs of the digestive system. In addition, a meal that is eaten leisurely instead of gulped tends to be more psychologically satisfying, a major step in learning to savor foods that are good for you.*

## SHE FAVORS SWEETS WITH MORE SUBSTANCE

Nina Hanson didn't even realize she had a sugar problem until she was 40 years old and taking a weekend trip to Maine with her boyfriend. "We'd stopped in Troy, New York, for our favorite treat, a hot-fudge sundae," she says. "About 20 minutes later, I suddenly became very anxious and physically miserable. My boyfriend became frantic, saying that I was acting like an old girlfriend who had hypoglycemia."

The couple stopped at a health food store in Burlington, Vermont, where the owner told Nina about hidden sugar in food and advised her to eliminate sugar and junk items from her diet. "That evening, I ate fish and steamed vegetables, salad without dressing, and tea instead of my usual coffee and cream," says Nina, who lives in Bridgeport, New York. "By the next morning, I was feeling more myself again. By the end of the day, I felt much calmer than I ever remembered being in my life."

Nina was later tested and discovered that she did indeed have hypoglycemia, so she started paying more attention to everything she ate. Her big breakthrough came when she learned about the glycemic index (GI) in Dr. Andrew Weil's book *Eating Well for Optimum Health*. "When foods have more fiber in them, the body takes longer to break them down, thereby slowing the absorption of sugar and starch into the bloodstream," she says.

Dr. Weil mentioned that fruits with a GI of less than 55 would provide the body with energy over a longer period of time and help ease hunger pangs. "Looking through his book, I found a number of fruits with low glycemic numbers and thus more fiber: apples, apricots, cherries, grapefruit, peaches, pears, and plums," says Nina.

"I noticed that I especially needed to get my blood sugar stabilized when I got home from work, because I was anxious and either craved food or had no appetite," Nina continues. "To test Dr. Weil's theory, I bought several low-glycemic fruits and ate one either when I left work or when I arrived home. I found that my blood sugar stabilized after about 5 minutes and stayed that way for about half an hour before I got anxious or craved junk food again. At that point, I had to either eat another piece of fruit or make myself a sugar-free meal." Still, she could plan for a nutritious dinner, rather than just inhaling everything in sight.

"Once I got off sugar at age 40, I realized that I probably would have been a lot calmer had I known about sugar sooner and had I not started bingeing on junk food and soda when I was a teen," says Nina, now 51. "My emotions and my attitude in life are so different now. I feel more secure, less frantic, more centered, and much happier."

### WINNING ACTION

**Make sure your sweets include fiber.** Perhaps it's not possible for every sweet you eat to have fiber, but you *should make an effort to choose foods that provide your body with more than empty calories. If you like to start the morning with a sweetened cold cereal, for example, try sugar-coated shredded wheat instead of a chocolate variety. And choose fruits like apples, grapefruit, pears, and plums instead of candy bars. These fruits may be more expensive than candy, but you'll need to eat less of them to feel fuller. And you'll reap the benefits of both the fiber and the nutrients fruits contain.*

## *SHE KEEPS HER SWEETS HIDDEN AWAY*

Paula Giovino knows she can't resist a chocolate bar or a half-eaten cake lying in plain sight on her kitchen counter. "If it's in front of me, I'll pick at it all day long," she says. But stash her sweets in the pantry, she's less likely to be tempted.

For Paula, who's 38 and lives in Freeport, New York, out of sight really does mean out of mind. "Right now, I still have three blocks of chocolate from an 18-inch Belgian chocolate bar in a Ziploc bag in my cabinet," she says proudly. "And I've had them there for 2 years."

Hiding sweets is a family tradition she inherited from her mother, a health food fanatic who rarely fed her children sweets. Once a month, she'd buy a treat, and Paula and her sister would comb the house looking for it. "One time, in ninth grade, my sister leaned against the dishwasher, accidentally turning it on, and we just let it run," Paula recalls. "But when we opened it, we found a soggy box of Ring Dings."

Growing up with limited sweets turned Paula into a sugarholic.

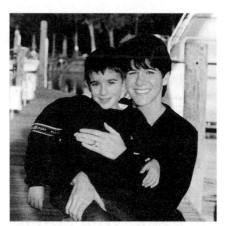

After her son Justin was born, Paula had even more reason to keep sweets out of the house.

At her worst, she could devour four doughnuts in a single sitting or half a tray of brownies at a time, especially when she had PMS. All that began to change in 1994 , when she got pregnant. Paula decided that she wasn't going to eat sweets during her pregnancy, and she wouldn't feed them to her son either. "Everything I read just said sugar wasn't good for kids, and I was concerned that sugar could cause overactive behavior," she says.

Paula knew she had to set a good example if she wanted to keep her son, Justin, away from sweets. So she stopped buying sugary foods and keeping them in her house. She started snacking on fruit, yogurt, and raisins coated with natural sugar from grains and fruit. She also began using cookbooks with sugar-free recipes and adapted her favorite muffin and brownie recipes by using date sugar instead of white sugar, a trick she picked up from her mother. Now, when Justin goes to a birthday party, Paula brings along a piece of special sugar-free cake.

These days, Paula still has sugar cravings at certain times of the month, but she usually grabs a piece of fruit. Occasionally, she allows herself to enjoy a brownie or a cannoli—but only when Justin is out of sight. And just to make sure she's got it under control, Paula still hides any sweets that get into the house. "If it's hidden away, I won't eat it," she says. "I can even survive something from the bakery if it's in a box and tied up with a string."

## WINNING ACTION

**Hide forbidden foods.** *If you can't keep them out of the house entirely, at least keep sugary temptations out of view. You'll forget they're even around. Going one step further, you may want to ask any family members with a sweet tooth to enjoy their treats in another room, where you can't see them and be tempted. Be sure to keep plenty of nutritious, naturally sweet snacks on hand—a bowl of fruit on the kitchen counter, for example—for those moments when you've just got to have something to eat.*

# SHE CREATED HER OWN SUGAR-FREE SNACKS

When summer rolls around and temperatures rise, most people head to the refrigerator to cool off with an ice cream sandwich or Popsicle. But not Janice Saeger, of Emmaus, Pennsylvania.

Oh, she heads to the refrigerator, all right—but she has a special treat waiting of her own concoction: frozen fruit pops with no sugar added. "I love melon, so when I have the time, I throw watermelon or cantaloupe (or other fruit) into the blender and make frozen pops, sometimes adding a little juice to the mix," she says. "Sugar-free Popsicles have a bitter taste I don't like, so I'd rather make my own."

At age 51, Janice is finding it a little more difficult to lose weight, but she's determined to do so, especially since she was recently diagnosed with high blood pressure. She already maintains an exercise program and hardly ever drinks soda, so she decided that the snacks—"the Doritos and Fritos and chocolate candy, anything chocolate"—had to go.

While her homemade juice pops serve as a great snack substitute in the summertime, melons become scarce or expensive when the weather turns cold—which meant Janice had to create another snack for herself.

After checking out health food stores, she put together a combination of soy nuts, raw almonds, yogurt-covered raisins, and dried fruit. The dried fruit—primarily figs, apricots, and pineapple—contains no added sugar, and combined with the yogurt raisins, it gives the mix a sweet taste.

The mix satisfies Janice's desire for something sweet, fatty, and crunchy all at the same time, and she keeps containers of the mix both at work and at home. "This is redirecting my desire," she says. "It's tricking me into snacking on something that's good. It works for me."

### W I N N I N G   A C T I O N

**Make your own sugar-free snacks.** *You needn't resign yourself to eating whatever packaged, processed sweets you find in the supermarket. And you needn't even rely on whatever sugar-free products are available. You can create your own juice combos, shakes, frozen pops, fruit-nut mixes, and more with common ingredients* *from the supermarket, health food store, or farmers' market. With a little experimentation, you're sure to come up with homemade sugarless treats that you'll love. If you want to try Janice's snack mix, keep in mind that yogurt-covered raisins may be sweetened with sugar. Also, dried fruit is very calorie-dense, so monitor your portion sizes.*

## HE ATTACKS HIS CRAVINGS WITH AN AMINO ACID

In 1996, coming off a self-imposed sugar-restricted diet, Noah Scales started downing sweets obsessively. "I found I couldn't stop myself," he recalls.

An amateur chef, he spent hours in the kitchen, creating his own recipes for candy. He searched for the perfect combination of sugar and peanut butter, tossing in ingredients like cinnamon and butter—and even pureed chickpeas, tofu, and whey powder, for creaminess. He'd eat about a fifth of his recipes, then throw out the rest.

Back then, Noah, a Web page designer from Santa Cruz, California, craved sugar all day long. Powerfully. By exercising daily, he managed to maintain a stable weight, between 150 and 160 pounds on his 6-foot frame. Nevertheless, in 1998, he began to experience feelings of hopelessness. "I was embarrassed about the way I was eating. Whenever my housemates saw me, I was in the kitchen," he says.

In December 1999, still bingeing regularly on peanut butter and sugar, though in smaller amounts, Noah went to a doctor. Noah suggested that he try restricting his sugar intake to less than 50 grams a day, and his doctor agreed. To start, whenever he felt a craving, he'd reach for fruit instead of a sweet.

Noah quickly found this was no piece of cake and soon returned to his doctor. "I told her this was just too big a sugar craving for me to handle," he says. At that point, his doctor suggested that Noah take glutamine supplements.

Glutamine is one of 20 amino acids in the body. Noah found that a daily supplement tempered his otherwise fierce cravings. "I started at 5 grams, but that didn't make a dent, so my doctor recommended 5 more," he says. To counteract glutamine's suspected constipating effect, he also eats 40 grams of fiber a day.

Noah, who's now 27, has managed to limit sugar to less than 50 grams per day since early 2000. He no longer keeps sugar or sugar-laden foods in his house. He confesses that his low-sugar diet often leaves him feeling deprived. Still, he's pleased to be able to keep at bay those intense sugar urges that have plagued him since childhood.

### W I N N I N G   A C T I O N

***Try glutamine supplements.*** *If you feel dogged by an insatiable sweet tooth, you may want to check out glutamine. Supplements of the amino acid have been used to reduce cravings for alcohol; some people believe they may also reduce cravings for sugar and carbohydrates (though little research supports this claim). Although glutamine is considered safe in supplement form, be sure to check with your doctor before taking it, especially if you have liver or kidney problems.*

# SHE CONTROLS HER SWEET TOOTH WITH SUGAR-FREE MIXES

Missy Foy used to greet the morning with a soda.

"For me to drink eight or nine sodas in one day was nothing," she says. "My friends made fun of me and said that I should own stock in Sprite."

In the afternoon, she indulged in cookies—a box at a time. "Then I put the empty box in another person's trash can so no one would know who ate them," she says.

Those days are over. A diagnosis of type 1, or insulin-dependent, diabetes put an end to them.

Missy is a marathon runner, pounding out 110 miles a week from mid-February through early June and from September through December. She never worried about what she ate, figuring the exercise would negate any ill effects from sugar, fat, and salt. But when she learned at age 31 that she had diabetes, the diagnosis put an end to her love affair with soda.

"A sugar habit is hard to break," says Missy, who's 37 and lives in Durham, North Carolina. "But I didn't have a choice. Now, if I eat too much sugar, I feel really bad, like I'm drugged with a narcotic."

To satisfy her still-active sweet tooth, Missy turns to sugar-free powders—those used to make gelatin, fruit drinks, and cocoa, for example. She sprinkles them over plain yogurt and nuts for mid-morning snacks.

"There are a lot of sugar-free powders that taste pretty good," she says. "Be creative in how you use them."

Missy lost no weight after eliminating sugar from her diet. At 5 feet 6½ inches and 115 pounds, she didn't need to. But avoiding sugar keeps her blood sugar under control and makes her more energetic mentally.

"I am just more ready to take things on," she says. "If there is something I have to do, I just do it. I don't stop and debate whether I should wait. I even get something as basic as housework done when it needs doing."

Even so, it is difficult for her to think of her diabetes as a blessing. "It is a lot of work to keep diabetes under control," she says. "I can't ever take a day off."

Nevertheless, she adds, "I like the self-enlightenment that I have now. I know exactly how my body reacts to everything I give it."

### WINNING ACTION

***Use sugar-free powders to flavor snacks.*** *Sugar-free powders are what you buy to make flavored gelatin, fruit drinks like Kool-Aid, cocoa, iced tea, cheesecakes, and puddings. Certainly, you can use them as intended by following the package directions. But for more creative snacks and desserts, mix the powders with other ingredients. Combine fruity powders with nonfat cream cheese to get a satisfying sweet spread without extra calories. Sprinkle cocoa powder over cinnamon toast. Mix iced tea powder with a squirt of lemon juice and stir it into cut fruit for an exotic taste treat. And turn plain yogurt into a fabulous dessert by stirring in some cheesecake mix or pudding mix—think chocolate, lemon, even banana.*

# *TO BLOCK CRAVINGS, SHE REACHES FOR THE GREENS*

Debra Hockenberry's family had a bad history with blood sugar, one that she's inherited. "I've had tests showing my blood sugar level is very sensitive to the amount of sugar in my diet," says the Allentown, Pennsylvania, resident. "I also have low blood pressure. So if I eat too much sugar, my blood sugar gets out of balance, my eyesight goes bad, my feet and my hands become numb, and my concentration is completely affected."

Still, there were times when she gave in to temptation. "You may be aware that sugar is not a good thing," says Debra, age 40. "Yet it's almost habitual that you say, 'I can't stand it anymore. I'm going to have this Mounds bar.'" Unfortunately, for Debra, one candy bar per day all too often jumped to two, then three. "All of a sudden, the numbness, the inability to concentrate, the hunger pangs—all of it returned, because of the sugar high."

In the mid-1990s, though, a friend offered Debra an unusual suggestion for combating sugar cravings: Eat a salad instead. "I thought, 'That's the last thing I want,'" says Debra.

But she tried eating salads or other vegetables in place of sweets. To her surprise, she found that it works—"as long as I get my mind to focus on what's really going to help instead of automatically popping sugar," she says. "I try to be aware that this is a sugar craving and try to have something green. It satisfies the cravings so much more."

Besides helping to control her sweet tooth, this technique helps Debra maintain her weight. "I'm 5 feet 6 inches tall and usually weigh about 125 pounds," she says. "But I can easily go up to around 140 if I don't stay focused."

Debra has also noticed a correlation between the amount of

greens in her diet and the strength of her sugar cravings. When cravings start to bother her, that's a reminder to check how many greens she's getting each day.

Of course, sometimes—like when she's at work—"I may not be able to find a salad somewhere or have greens around," says Debra. In those circumstances, she meets her greens requirement by taking supplements that contain greens like chlorella, barley grass, spinach leaf, brussels sprouts, cabbage, and more. "I find if I take two in the morning and two in the afternoon, that's all I need for a complete day without sugar fixes," she says. "If I only take two in the morning, it helps throughout the day, but in the evening, I might start to want sugar or get cravings or hunger pangs more than usual.

"I don't know how this works, but it's something physical for me," says Debra. "They do what's necessary to keep that physical sensation away that I have during a sugar craving."

## WINNING ACTION

**Turn to greens to turn off sugar binges.** Keep the refrigerator stocked with an assortment of greens and other vegetables. Reach for these healthy items when you feel a sugar craving coming on. They may help fill you up, so you don't have room for the candy bars or chocolate cookies! And they're so low in calories you can eat all you want.

# *THESE SUBSTITUTES TAUGHT HIM A LESSON*

In his youth, Bryan Diamond was an exercise fiend, practicing martial arts and running up to 9 miles a day. "I could eat a whole chocolate cake in one night and not gain a pound," he says. "My metabolism burned right through it."

But in 1984, the same year he got married, he was involved in a car accident. The doctors told him to give up those activities to ease the stress on his knees, which had been injured in the accident. The forced absence of serious exercise didn't stop Bryan from hitting the sweets, however. "I was a serious chocoholic," he says. "If I went one night without sugar, it was a miracle."

Bryan's weight ballooned up over the years, eventually reaching more than 300 pounds. In mid-2000, his doctor diagnosed him with borderline diabetes and ordered him to exercise and lose some weight. He started riding a bike, only to be struck by a car during one of his workouts in October of that year—again halting the exercise and kicking the diabetes into full gear. "That's when everything changed," he says.

His diet went through a complete transformation: Breakfast became a special shake created especially for people with diabetes. In place of regular chocolate, Bryan discovered a candy bar containing a sugar substitute that tastes just like the real thing. "I have one every couple of nights, and that seems to reduce the cravings," he says. As for carbohydrates like bread and pasta (foods that most people with diabetes must monitor closely), "I replaced them with meat, poultry, eggs, and vegetables," he notes

He also found a yogurt shop near his home in Encino, California, that makes a sugar-free, fat-free frozen yogurt. "It's wonderful," says Bryan. "It tastes like real ice cream, but there's no sugar in it."

Just a few months into his low-sugar diet, this 36-year-old dropped from 320 pounds to 300 on his 6-foot-1 frame—and Bryan expects to drop much more now that he's discovered sugar-free treats. "It's almost like giving up smoking, where you have to replace the habit with something else," he says from experience. "To be honest, quitting sweets has been a little harder."

Harder, maybe, but Bryan is happy with the changes he's seen. "Before, I didn't have much energy and would be down a lot, almost like I was in a deep depression and didn't realize it," he says. "My body is feeling better now."

*W I N N I N G   A C T I O N*

**Find a sugar-free substitute for each sweet you crave.**
*Search the supermarkets for items that mimic the desired food as much as possible, except for the sugar content. Over time, you'll train your body to replace the desire for a particular sugar-laden booby trap with something healthier. This process won't happen overnight, but eventually, you'll change the unhealthy habits of your past and forge a new low-sugar future.*

# HE SAVES THE BEST FOR LAST

Not long ago, Richard Kirchknopf was a regular at the office vending machine, where he'd snack on Twinkies, brownies, and sugary tarts filled with pecans or raisins. To tame his sweet tooth—and counteract the weight gain it caused—he went on a low-carbohydrate diet and learned to eat his daily sweet at the end of the day, as the grand finale at supper. By saving his indulgence and limiting his carbohydrate intake, Richard no longer has daylong sugar cravings—nor an extra 40 pounds on his 6-foot frame.

Richard, 44, a computer programmer who lives in Toronto, used to nosh all day long. Drinking six cans of Coke in a day was nothing unusual, and he spent his nights gorging on sweets. "I'd eat a huge meal and still want desserts. The refrigerator used to have a revolving door," he jests.

In an attempt to be more healthy, Richard tried eating more fruits such as apples and strawberries, only to find he could eat large amounts of those, too. "I tried to redirect my craving to healthier sweets, but I was still losing the battle," he says.

Richard's weight topped out at 276 pounds before he tried *The Carbohydrate Addict's LifeSpan Program*. The plan calls for eating mostly vegetables and proteins, with just one starchy carbohydrate, preferably at the end of the day. The carbohydrate can be anything you choose, be it bread or pasta, cake or brownies. But it should be the last thing eaten after a low-carb meal—for example, right behind a large salad, a protein food, and a vegetable.

For Richard, the plan has meant skipping breakfast (which most nutrition experts don't recommend) and eating an early lunch, with just a salad and some ham or turkey. He also drinks a lot of water throughout the day and quit the Cokes cold turkey.

After 10 months on the diet, Richard lost 37 pounds. He felt more energetic, and his asthma symptoms improved, too. "I finally found something that has controlled my cravings," he says. "Before, I felt totally helpless, and my weight kept going up year after year."

Best of all, the plan allows Richard to still enjoy the sweets he loves. For his nightly carbohydrate, he generally prefers a sweet treat such as a chocolate bar or pastry, which he eats with a banana and milk. Now that he's maintaining his weight, when a tempting sweet appears earlier in the day, he simply packs it up and takes it home for dinner.

"Life without occasional sweets is impossible," he says. "Now, I know if I have cravings, I can always have something at supper. And supper is always less than 24 hours away."

### W I N N I N G   A C T I O N

**Limit your sweets to once a day.** *And fill up on vegetables and lean protein before you indulge. That way, you'll be less likely to overdo when you're ready to savor your special treat. Cutting back the rest of the time helps keep your cravings from taking over but still allows you to enjoy something sweet every day. Knowing you can indulge your sweet tooth on a controlled basis keeps binges from happening. But don't use this as license to eat as much sugar as you want. Resolve to keep the portion size just large enough to satisfy your desire for the sweet.*

# HE GIVES HIS CRAVINGS THE BRUSH-OFF

When W. Eric Martin was growing up, he never thought twice about the amount of sugar he ate. "I usually bought cookies and milk for lunch in the school cafeteria," he says. "Then when I got home from school, I'd drink a glass or two of soda and eat cookies nonstop while I watched cartoons. My mom made great cookies."

Eric's mother almost always had a homemade dessert ready

after supper. While he welcomed the cakes, pies, brownies, and other treats, he says that a dozen years after moving out of his parents' house, he still feels the need to end every meal with something sweet. "No matter what I have for lunch or dinner, I want to have a dessert, even if it's something small like two gingersnap cookies," he says.

"At restaurants, it's even worse," Eric continues. "My wife will say that she'll split a dessert with me—but then she'll put her spoon down before we're even halfway through. That's good for her, but I'll go ahead and finish it all myself."

Luckily for him, Eric has found a tool that helps push his sugar cravings away for a few hours: his toothbrush. "I brushed my teeth before breakfast one morning and then noticed that the orange juice tasted terrible," he says. "Cereal, too. I couldn't even eat it until I rinsed my mouth a lot.

"Then I had something sweet after brushing one night and that tasted terrible, too," says the 33-year-old Blackstone, Massachusetts, resident. Once that happened, he realized that he could easily avoid succumbing to sugar cravings in the future as long as he had a toothbrush with him. "The only thing that tastes okay after brushing is cold water," he says.

Eric is quick to point out that he doesn't necessarily brush each time he has a sugar craving. "It depends on how I feel about what else I've eaten that day," he explains.

Although Eric admits to putting on a few pounds since 1996, when he first began brushing away cravings, he says weight hasn't been a big concern for him. "I don't worry about getting fat as much as putting my body through the constant ups and downs that come with consuming too much sugar," he says. "I've learned to treat my body better and keep it running on an even keel by avoiding massive quantities of sweets.

*WINNING ACTION*

**When a sugar craving hits, reach for your toothbrush.**
*In fact, don't even wait for the craving to arrive. As soon as you finish your meal—whether it's in your dining room or at a restaurant—head for the bathroom and brush your teeth. Since a travel-size toothbrush and tube of toothpaste fit almost anywhere, it should be easy to carry your sugar-fighting tools wherever you go. Some toothpaste brands contain sugar or saccharin, though, so be sure to check the label before you buy lest they add fuel to your craving.*

# HE CULTIVATED A TASTE FOR SALTY AND SOUR FOODS

For almost two decades, Earl Moyer struggled to get sugar out of his life. It wasn't until he started eating more salty and sour foods that he was able to stamp out cravings for sweets.

Earl, who's 55 and lives in Rensselaer, New York, became interested in the subject of sugar in 1982, when he was diagnosed with diabetes. His own research convinced him that processed sugars had contributed to his illness.

"My addiction was so bad that one day I downed half a watermelon, 2 liters of Coke, and half a gallon of ice cream all in a couple of hours," he says. "I used to put 4 to 5 teaspoons of sugar in my tea. I think I may have broken a record in New York state for having the highest blood sugar level when it went over a thousand."

The seeds of his sugar addiction were sown in his youth. Earl's father worked in a bakery, and the family often ate baked goods for breakfast and lunch. As an adult, Earl worked as an actor and spent a lot of time on the run. "I would eat doughnuts for breakfast and peanut butter and jelly sandwiches for lunch," he says. "I was grabbing snacks like candy bars all the time, and I drank a lot of soda."

All the sugar made for a lot of fatigue, and Earl slept as much as 12 hours a night. When he was diagnosed with diabetes, he made the decision to stop eating sugar. But meaningful change took years. "It was a real process," he says. "I would slip several times just like with any addiction."

The more he learned about processed sugar, the more militant he became. At one point, he even wanted to do a documentary on the subject. "I'd be grabbing candy bars out of babies' hands. I wanted to save the world from this evil," he says.

To save himself, Earl began eating more salty and sour foods. Pickles, sauerkraut, and popcorn became regular staples in his diet. He also used a lot of salsa, mustard, and sesame oil in his foods. "These foods took away the cravings for sweets," he says. "I began to taste how sweet a pear is. I began to taste how sweet an apple is. I could even taste the sweetness in brown rice and other grains."

Earl also cut out most refined carbohydrates and took up swimming and walking. At the same time, he became more spiritual, a development that only fueled his conviction that what he ate was critical to his well-being. "As my spirituality grew, I realized my body really is a temple, and what I put in it matters," he says.

These days, Earl rarely eats processed sugars and now needs only half the amount of insulin that he was originally taking. "I used to feel tired and sluggish all the time," he says. "Now, I feel a lot more energetic. It's like a new life." He is working on a book about sugar addictions that he is calling *SOS—Stay Off Processed Sugars: A Plea from a Diabetic.*

### WINNING ACTION

**Add more salty and sour foods to your diet.** Eating these kinds of foods will sensitize your taste buds to the sweetness in sugary foods. You may find that most sweets are simply too cloying. And that can help you appreciate the sweetness in natural foods like fruits, vegetables, and even grains. In addition, salty and sour foods are inherently low in sugar, so you're not simply switching your sugar intake from one food group to another. If you've got high blood pressure, however, check with your doctor before adding more salty items to your diet.

## SHE FOUND THAT RAW FOOD SUITS HER BETTER

"I was a complete sugarholic," says Carole Myers of Los Angeles. But the biggest problem with her sugar addiction was that she *didn't* gain weight, so she was unaware that sugar was causing any problem.

"I had suffered from migraines since I was a kid and couldn't eat when I was ill," she says. Her eating habits mirrored a bulimic's in that she seesawed back and forth from not eating at all to bingeing once the pain cleared. And the food Carole did eat came from a nutritionist's nightmare: Breakfast might be potato sticks, dip, and chocolate milk; lunch would be a box of chocolate chip cookies and whipped cream.

Carole's migraines plagued her into adulthood. "I'd start each morning with Excedrin and then take other, prescription drugs throughout the day to compensate for the Excedrin," she says. "I was able to run long distances, look pretty good, and still be incredibly ill—but I was so anesthetized that I didn't know how sick I really was."

She also developed rheumatoid arthritis, an autoimmune disease in which a person's immune system attacks healthy tissue as if it were a foreign invader. "I had it so severely that at one point I had a handicapped sticker on the car," she says.

When a chiropractor gave Carole a book that suggested sugar might be behind the rheumatoid arthritis (although no research supports this theory), she decided she could try cutting out sweets for a short while. To her surprise, she says, "when I stopped eating candy and cake and the obvious sugars, my pain started going away."

But it didn't go away completely, so Carole took a closer look at her diet. Convinced that it was doing her harm, she decided to switch to raw foods. There were difficulties at first—"You just don't know what to eat," says Carole—but since 1994, she's become more knowledgeable about how to follow a healthy raw diet. Now, breakfast might be brown rice soaked overnight and cold-pressed olive oil, and dinner will be raw fish or sprouted beans. "In between meals, I might eat bananas, presoaked nuts and seeds, fresh vegetable juice drinks, salads, or raw milk. Believe it or not, it's all delicious," she says.

"My diet is a radical change," admits Carole, who will soon be a first-time grandmother. "Today, I have no migraines and no arthritis and take no medicine. I'm the healthiest and happiest I've ever been."

*WINNING ACTION*

**Eat more raw foods.** *You might not want to switch completely to uncooked foods, but you can incorporate lots of raw fruits and vegetables—even soaked grains—into your diet. Muesli, a mixture of soaked oats and fruit, makes a filling breakfast. Salads are always good for hearty lunches and dinners and can be much more complex than a handful of greens. Most vegetables are excellent raw, and their fiber is very filling. Further, it takes more effort to eat raw foods, so you have time to become satisfied and are less likely to automatically reach for a sugary treat to finish off the meal.*

# SHE SNACKS WELL NOW TO STOP UNCONTROLLED NIBBLING LATER

When Tara Cranmer arrived home from work, she was hungry and ready to eat. Since she prefers to have dinner later in the evening, she snacked on junk food—including sweets like chocolate and cookies—to tide her over until mealtime.

Once dinner was over, Tara invariably ended up downing another sweet or two. "I would graze all evening long while watching TV," says the 30-year-old resident of Macungie, Pennsylvania. "Dinner was surrounded by a lot of junk food. And I wouldn't stop when I wasn't hungry anymore."

Tara had always been super skinny growing up. "I could eat as much as I wanted without gaining an ounce—until I hit age 25 and it caught up with me," she says. Once she noticed she was putting on a few extra pounds, she began to examine her lifelong eating habits more closely. "It was really frustrating that I'd always been able to eat whatever I wanted and all of a sudden I couldn't," she says.

Realizing her evening-long grazing started as soon as she got home, Tara decided to make those first snacks more filling than her usual fare. "I would have a piece of bread with peanut butter on it or a couple of pretzels with juice—something healthier than sweets," she says. "Then I didn't need to start on the junk food."

With her new dietary strategy, which she launched in the spring of 2000, Tara still has something sweet, usually chocolate, after dinner. But, she says, "I don't feel I need so many sweets because I'm not eating them on an empty stomach anymore."

Tara, who is 5 feet 3 inches tall, lost about 3 pounds just by cutting back on her evening sweets. Breaking the sugar habit was hard, she says, yet a mere 2 weeks after she changed her diet, she found she could satisfy her sugar cravings with far less. "There was a time when I felt like I needed to be doing something while I watched TV because I was so used to having a snack in my hands, but I just set my mind against grazing on sweets," she says. "If you can get through those first 2 weeks, then you've got a pretty good shot."

## WINNING ACTION

***Choose a sensible predinner snack.*** *When you get home from work and start looking for something to tide you over until dinner, don't reach for a handful of cookies and a glass of soda—or else you'll be headed for seconds as soon as the meal ends. Instead of choosing sweets, pick up something that's a little more nutritious and filling, maybe a protein snack bar or peanut butter or* *cheese on crackers. You may consume as many calories as you used to before dinner, but you're less likely to get carried away snacking later on.*

## SHE TAKES HER SUGAR BY THE DROP

To clear up a recurring health problem, Erica Diamond had to make some tough nutritional choices. "On my doctor's recommendation, I gave up all sugar and all fruit," she says.

Out went the sweet rolls and ice cream that she loved, along with most of the other snacks that she ate. In came a new, disciplined outlook toward eating. "It's hard to say no to birthday cakes, wedding cakes, and desserts when people are asking you to try something," she says—but she found the strength to turn those treats aside.

Of course, Erica couldn't just eliminate food from her diet without something taking its place, so she searched the supermarket aisles for nonsugary snacks. She found salt-free chips and a low-sodium salsa (since she had also cut back on sodium), and she started getting more into vegetables.

"My doctor said that I should find things I can chew because the body likes to chew," says Erica, who lives in Encino, California. "So I buy little peeled carrots and find interesting things to dip them in. I've gotten to the point where they taste sweet."

The 49-year-old also liked to snack on plain, unsweetened yogurt, but she couldn't figure out how to sweeten it to make it more palatable. "Then a friend suggested that she try adding a combination of slivered almonds, cinnamon, and a little liquid stevia—a sugar substitute.

"What I found with the new snacks was that I didn't have to eat as much. Smaller portions would satisfy me," says Erica. "When I eat carbohydrates or sugar, I just can't get enough. These other items satisfy my urge to chew." That includes snacks such as unsalted raw almonds, cashews, and pistachios. "They have some bulk to them, so they're also satisfying."

Since Erica started her sugar-free diet in January 2001, her symptoms have vanished, along with 40 pounds—and she doesn't see herself returning to her old eating habits anytime soon. "I don't look at this as a diet but as a lifestyle change," she says. "I can choose to be healthy or choose to stay sick." After living both ways, the choice is easy.

## WINNING ACTION

***Use liquid stevia in place of sugar.*** *Stevia, which is sold as a dietary supplement, comes from a South American shrub and has been used as a sweetening agent for centuries. The most abundant component of the leaves, stevioside, is 150 to 250 times as sweet as sugar and, best of all, noncaloric. Stevia is available in the form of powdered leaves, liquid extract, or purified stevioside. The liquid version can be used as an easy, sweet addition to your coffee, tea, yogurt, or iced tea without the worry of added calories. For more ideas on its use, ask the clerks at your health food store or search for recipes on the Internet and at bookstores.*

# *SHE BUYS TREATS THAT SHE CAN'T EAT*

Sweets were never a problem for Jeanie Stout as a child. "I was brought up poor, and often we didn't have enough good food to eat," she says. "I was extremely skinny as a kid."

That all changed once she married. "I got my own kitchen and learned to love to cook for my husband and me. And I grew in size," says Jeanie, who favored cakes, cookies, and sweet breads.

Eventually, Jeanie realized what was happening to her and decided she couldn't go on like she had in the past. "I knew it was healthier to reduce sugar in my diet," she says. "So I started to experiment with my favorite recipes by cutting the sugar in half. When it called for a cup of sugar, I used half a cup."

When that worked out, this resident of Moravian Falls, North Carolina, started finding ways of forgoing sugar altogether and choosing other treats that would satisfy her. "If I'm out shopping and think I need a sugary snack, I buy myself something just as satisfying instead of food," she says. "Maybe a new flavor of decaf tea, a good book to read, flowers, earrings, or some pretty new thing to wear in my hair."

Clothing is another "sweet" treat, one that helps Jeanie focus on her diet at the same time she improves her wardrobe. "I buy something pretty for a special occasion that's already planned, and I look forward to wearing it," she says. "If I gain weight, I won't be able to fit into it.

"Once I stopped by a fudge shop just to smell the fudge, but I didn't buy or even taste anything. So I decided to reward myself by splurging on an article of clothing," Jeanie continues. "It was a size smaller than what I had been wearing, a medium instead of a large. That made me happy. I put it away for a trip to the beach that was planned for about 4 weeks later. I knew I had to stay the same weight to fit into it."

And unlike a sweet that she can use only once, Jeanie's treats come into play again and again to help her avoid sugar. "I try to make myself look lovely before going shopping or eating out," says Jeanie, who's now 42. "Depending on the time I have, I put on a bit of makeup and wear nice, neat clothes. If I feel good about my appearance, I care more about myself and can more quickly avoid self-destructive habits."

### W I N N I N G   A C T I O N

**Find new treats to replace the sweets.** *Sure, chocolate and brownies taste great—but within a minute, the flavor is gone, and all you're left with are the calories. Instead of spending money on ephemeral pleasures, look around for treats that you'll enjoy on a more permanent basis: maybe a new book or video that you can turn to whenever you crave sweets, a deck of cards to keep your hands busy, or a new CD that will have you dancing around the house instead of stuck in the kitchen. The possibilities are endless.*

## SHE SUITED A TASTE FOR SUGAR TO A TEA

After dinner, as the day winds to a close, it hits. "That is our worst time for craving sweets," says Linda Paist. "That is when we want cookies, ice cream, or cake with icing."

But she and her husband, Wistar, have found a way to control those sugar cravings. Not by ignoring them or by worrying them into going away but by—in the tiniest way—giving in to them.

"We each have a cup of tea with 2 teaspoons of sugar in it," says Linda, who's 40 and lives in Breinigsville, Pennsylvania. "It cuts down on the craving for sweets and has a whole lot less sugar than a candy bar."

Both Paists are trying to lose weight. Linda, at 5 feet 3 inches, has lost about 5 pounds in 5 months and weighs 122. She wants to get down to 115. Her husband, who is 47 years old and 5 feet 6 inches tall, weighs 185. His goal is 170, a figure to which he got 12 pounds closer over the course of a year.

"Drinking tea was one of the things he did," Linda says. "Whereas before we would have ice cream or a handful of Double Stuf Oreos, now we have tea."

Linda says that it is the combination of hot liquid and sweetness that, strangely, satisfies. Any kind of tea works, she says, from the old standbys to trendy herbal teas. Coffee dressed up with a sweet flavored cream also works, she says.

Not that ignoring chocolate fudge ice cream is always easy, even over tea. "Sometimes, it takes two cups of tea to work," Linda admits. "But even that is better than eating a big piece of cake."

She says that it is not just the taste of sweet foods that attracts but the emotions we associate with them. "It is a comfort kind of thing," she says. "When I was growing up, we usually had Jell-O or pudding for dessert. But for special occasions, we had a fancy dessert. And when we visited my grandmother, I would sit on the couch with her and we would eat ice cream and watch Lawrence Welk. It made me feel good."

Linda also has cravings for sweets at midday. On the rare occasions she can't fight them off, she allows herself to have a piece of chocolate—or caramel-flavored hard candy. That tides her over until she can get home to her new comfort food: tea.

### W I N N I N G   A C T I O N

**Let sweetened tea stave off sugar cravings.** *What could be a better replacement for sugary comfort food than a warm cup of the liquid Grandma used to make? Although tea is commonly sweetened with sugar, it's a lot less than you'd find in a piece of chocolate cake or whatever other high-calorie indulgence you'd normally reach for. There's an almost endless variety of teas available. At night, try a decaffeinated variety or herbal tea. Sweetened fruit tea, such as a berry tea, is especially good. And as you continue in this new habit, gradually lessen the amount of sugar you put in the tea—eventually, the tea alone might satisfy.*

# STASHING SWEETS IN THE FREEZER KEEPS TEMPTATION AT BAY

Marci David never considered herself a real sugar fiend. But she admits to a fondness for baked goods—which could spell trouble in her part-time job as a caterer. While she almost always has sweets in her house, she's learned to hide them in her basement freezer. That way, it's too much trouble to get to them. "I don't want to go into the basement barefoot," she explains.

Marci, 59, of Albany, New York, didn't eat a lot of sweets as a child, but she put away her fair share of baked goods in college.

Twice a week, she indulged in doughnuts at the dining hall. "By the middle of the morning, I would feel awful—tired, sluggish, and weak," she says. "I figured that out when I was 18 years old, but I still ate sweets because they tasted good."

Once out of college, Marci and her friends would pick up the *New York Times* at 2 A.M. Sunday mornings, then walk next door to the bakery, where fresh pastries were being prepared. "We'd bang on the door, and they'd let us in," she recalls. "Then we'd go back home and eat pastries while doing the crossword puzzle."

A runner, Marci noticed that her legs felt heavier and harder to lift on days after she had eaten sugar. She became concerned because her family had a history of diabetes, and she believed she might be hypoglycemic—a suspicion that was confirmed in the mid-1970s. On top of that, Marci had always struggled with her weight.

It wasn't until 1998 that she finally got serious about slimming down. She cut back on carbohydrates, added more protein, and ditched most sweets. Now, she eats vegetables and protein at every meal and snacks on almonds in between. To keep her mind off sweets, she learned to occupy herself with civic volunteer work, reading, and gardening. "You just have to decide on a strategy," she says.

Of course, Marci still has to contend with the baked goods that come with the catering territory. Even when she isn't on the job, she enjoys cooking for her friends. Sometimes, if she has a few hours to spare, she does her baking in advance and stores the goodies in the basement freezer—ready to go in case she gets busy or hosts a small party.

Having sweets in the house does make for temptation, but hiding them in the basement helps keep Marci away. The upstairs freezer just doesn't work. "The other day, I found a biscotti in there, and I ate it," she says.

Marci's diligence has paid off with a loss of 50 pounds from her 5-foot-5 frame. Now weighing 192, she wants to lose at least 25 more pounds. With help from her basement freezer, she's managed to put a freeze on her cravings for sweets—which should make her goal attainable.

## WINNING ACTION

**Make indulging inconvenient.** *If you must store sweets in your house, stash them where they're hard to get at. A freezer in the basement or garage is ideal. Getting to the basement or garage typically takes time to put on shoes—and maybe even a jacket in the middle of winter. Thawing the sweet provides just enough time for you to reconsider your actions and ask yourself if you really want the sugar.*

# A SHORT-TERM VEGAN DIET ERADICATED HER SWEET TOOTH

In the old days, Maria Salomão would swig a packet of sugar. But these days, she nearly gags when she sees how much of the sweet stuff is in food. A 3-month stint as a vegan turned the former sugar addict into someone who now tastes chemicals in ice cream.

Maria, the 34-year-old owner of a San Francisco public relations firm, grew up believing that sugar was a staple food, much like eggs and bread. She loved desserts, especially ice cream and chocolate cake, and ate sweets virtually every week.

In the mid-1990s, after Maria broke up with a boyfriend who

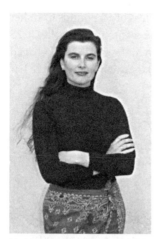

Maria says a short-term vegan diet changed her life—and her love of sweets.

loved to eat, her mother noticed that she had gained weight. Normally a size 6—she never steps on a scale—she had grown to a size 12.

That's when Maria, who had always been thin, decided to bone up on nutrition. "I read that foods you think are 'basic,' like sugar, really aren't basic at all," she says. "A child's love of Twinkies and Ho Hos, for instance, is an acquired taste."

Maria doesn't believe in dieting, so she decided to try veganism instead. That meant giving up all meats, poultry, and anything with eggs, milk, or sugar in it. "Bodywise, I felt so great," she says. "But every time I went to someone's house or a restaurant, I had to give my friends a laundry list of what I couldn't eat. And they'd crack, 'Oh, *you're* a lot of fun!'"

Eventually, after struggling to stick with her strict vegan lifestyle, Maria began drifting away from it. But it already had a profound effect on her tastes. Once, when she tried eating ice cream, "it didn't even taste like ice cream," she says. "It tasted like a chemical pool. Being vegan for a while had gotten rid of that sugar thing."

Maria was also distraught by news reports showing children in Third World countries toiling in sugar fields for low wages and under poor working conditions. The images remain with her even now, years later.

Nowadays, Maria eats a vegetarian diet that includes fish. She doesn't eat processed foods and instead consumes lots of fruits, nuts, tofu, and beans. She also took up yoga, meditation, and walking. And when she does get a sugar craving—usually when she's bored—she realizes it's a yen for a memory, not what the food actually tastes like. "If it's a really strong craving, I'll eat something sweet," she says. "But then I find it tastes terrible."

Without sugar, Maria feels more energetic. Her complexion is better, her hair more vibrant. "Going vegan really changed my life," she says. "You have only one body, and I'm determined to take care of mine. As one of my mentors, inspirational speaker Les Brown, says, 'You have to be willing to do the things today that others won't do, in order to have the things tomorrow that others won't have.'"

## WINNING ACTION

***Consider eating a vegan diet for a while.*** *It doesn't have to be a permanent change, but it may make you more sensitive to the sweetness of sugar. When you revert to a more liberal approach to eating, you'll be less likely to fall back into a sugar habit. Vegans do not eat any animal-based foods, including dairy products, eggs, and possibly even honey. According to a position paper from the American Dietetic Association, people who eat any form of vegetarian diet are generally at a lower risk for chronic degenerative diseases—such as heart disease, high blood pressure, and cancer—than nonvegetarians. If you decide to try a vegan diet, consider taking a supplement of vitamin $B_{12}$, which vegans tend to run low on.*

# *PEANUT BUTTER HITS HER SWEET SPOT*

For Ellen Navitsky, no meal was complete without dessert. Breakfast cereal was followed by a doughnut or Rice Krispies Treats. Her workplace cafeteria supplied an array of pies and baked goods to complete lunch. And dinner inevitably ended with hot chocolate and some kind of baked good.

"Unfortunately, I've passed this habit on to my 7-year-old son. After every meal, he asks for a snack. He's a little chubby for his age, so I'm trying to get him out of the habit of eating something sweet after every meal," says Ellen, 31, of Allentown, Pennsylvania.

That means teaching by example. Ellen gave up sweets twice before when she developed gestational diabetes during her pregnancies. But this time, she says, "It started as a Lenten sacrifice, first with chocolate, then with all desserts."

For the first few days, Ellen tried to forgo all sugar, but that tactic soon failed. "I hit a wall because I was dying for something sweet," she says. To compensate, she started looking for foods with intense flavors that lacked sugar. She had some success with oranges, flavored coffees, apples with cheese, and hard-boiled eggs with crackers, but her biggest sugar killer proved to be a food she had at first avoided: peanut butter.

"The big thing for me was cutting out fat, so I didn't eat peanut butter even though I love it," says Ellen. "Now, I'm finding that in moderation it's satisfying me, and I'm not snacking on sugary stuff."

Whereas Ellen used to eat Cocoa Puffs and Oreo O's for breakfast—sugared cereals purchased for her children—she now prefers plain oatmeal topped with a tablespoon of peanut butter and a little honey. She also enjoys a spoonful of peanut butter with an apple or banana. "Fruit on its own is boring to me," she says. "This satisfies me almost as much as a candy bar."

Not one for name brands, Ellen prefers the fresh-ground peanut butter sold in her grocery store and the all-natural variety available in the cafeteria at work. She makes a point of pouring off the oil that rises to the top. "It makes the peanut butter chunkier, and I like it better," she says.

So far, Ellen's new diet is working well. She doesn't crave lunch as early as she used to, and she doesn't tire so easily in the evenings. "I feel satisfied in what I've been doing," she says, "so there isn't a nagging feeling to go out and grab some candy and pie."

### W I N N I N G   A C T I O N

**Eat peanut butter to keep you full and reduce cravings.**
*With high-protein foods like peanut butter, you'll feel satisfied longer and be less likely to splurge between meals. An added benefit of peanut butter is that it contains healthy monounsaturated fat that can help lower your risks for heart disease and diabetes and may even help you lose weight. Limit yourself to about 2 tablespoons a day and subtract fat and calories elsewhere in your diet to compensate for what's in the peanut butter. If you don't like peanut butter, choose something else with protein and a little good fat, such as nuts, low-fat cheese, or a hard-boiled egg. Yes, these items contain fat—but so do doughnuts, pies, pastries, and ice cream, which accompany their fat with lots of sugar.*

# *HE TREATS HIS BODY WITH RESPECT, NOT SUGAR*

Russ Payne has prostate cancer. But the old cliché that he's "battling" his disease does not sit well with him.

"I have cancer cells in my body, and they do not belong there," he says. "I want them out, but my body is not a battleground. I try to keep things as peaceful as I can."

So Russ is learning to treat himself well. He has bought a hammock and spends time there with his favorite books. He plays banjo in a band that specializes in music from the 1940s. He rides his bicycle 10 miles three or four times a week and sails in the bay near his Long Neck, Delaware, home. And he eats no sweets.

"People ask me, 'Don't you cheat a little bit?' But who would I be cheating? Myself. I do this because it is good for me."

Russ, a 68-year-old telephone company retiree, was diagnosed with prostate cancer in 1997. As part of his treatment, he went to Hippocrates Health Institute, an alternative treatment center in West Palm Beach, Florida. There he was advised to cut back on sugar, which supplies only empty calories and causes a lot of stress to the body.

"I had always been very careful with what I ate, except for sugar," he says. "I enjoyed anything sweet. I could devour half a pie in one evening while watching TV, with no problem—or so I thought."

Those days are over. Russ stopped eating sugar as soon as he was told too much was bad for him. It hasn't been easy. After performances with his band, refreshments—usually ice cream and cake—are served. The cookie plate is passed.

He still gets hankerings for any kind of pie. "I was an indiscriminate pie eater," he says. "The other day, I saw someone eating a slice of cherry pie, and it looked so good."

But he finds it easy to resist when he reminds himself that doing so is good for him. "I just sit there and drink a glass of water," he says. "Either I'm going to control my body or my body is going to control me. I am learning to put myself first, and not eating sugar is good for me."

## WINNING ACTION

**Learn to be good to yourself.** *Many people choose to pamper themselves by indulging in a sweet treat to soothe a momentary desire. But truly being good to yourself means eating only foods that are healthy for you and that will make you feel good both physically and mentally. Once you understand that you are worth the extra effort required to resist a cookie or a piece of pie, doing so becomes easier.*

# HYPNOSIS EMPOWERED HIM TO MAKE BETTER DECISIONS

Rodger Farquhar used to go through half a bag of M&M's at a sitting. A whole sleeve of Oreos would disappear before bedtime.

He wanted to stop the sugar cravings that were directing his eating. At 5 feet 11 inches and 206 pounds, he wanted to lose weight. But after trying and failing, he realized that he needed some outside help.

"I saw a therapist," says Rodger, who's 50 and lives in Sarasota, Florida. "I used to like to have sugar every day: cookies, chocolate. Finally, I'm not craving big bags of M&M's."

Early in 2001, Rodger sought assistance from Elizabeth Bo-horquez, a clinical medical hypnotherapist at the Sarasota Medical Hypnosis Institute. He had two sessions with the hypnotist and now regularly listens to tapes that she gave him to reinforce the lessons he learned.

"She empowered me to make better decisions," Rodger says. "I learned the ability to say no, to not fall victim to cravings."

Through hypnosis, Rodger learned about the connection between what he eats and how he feels. "Elizabeth talked about the body as a garden and said that we should constantly try to weed out the bad things. It makes you think that your mind and body are closely connected."

Rodger says that within 3 months of undergoing hypnosis, he lost 6 pounds. But the scale doesn't tell the whole story. Because Roger has been lifting weights, much of the fat he was toting has been replaced by muscle.

In addition, his mental health has improved. "I have a more consistent level of temper," he says. "Sugar made me hyper. Now I am more calm and have fewer mood swings. And I feel more clear-headed."

Rodger's turnaround does not mean that sugary foods are out of his life forever. "I cheat a little bit about every 2 weeks," he says. "Just a little, something that is unforgettable. Now, I am able to stop with one cookie."

### WINNING ACTION

**Consider professional hypnosis.** *While some people do just fine with self-hypnosis techniques, others may need the help of a professional hypnotherapist. It's not a treatment that appeals to everyone, but the fact is, hypnosis has been* *used for centuries to modify human thoughts and behaviors. If you're prone to sugar binges, for example, a hypnotherapist can give you the suggestion that these binges are harming your body, so you no longer want sweets. To find a qualified practitioner in your area, ask your doctor or check with your local hospital's referral service.*

## MIND OVER MATTER HELPED HER CONQUER SUGAR

Carrie Havranek likens chocolate chip cookies to "a little devil sitting on my shoulder." But she has learned that a little distraction goes a long way in keeping the devil from climbing off her shoulder and into her mouth.

"If my fiancé is eating cookies, I just leave the room," says 27-year-old Carrie of Easton, Pennsylvania. "I pick up a magazine, clean up my office, any activity to get my mind off the cookie."

Her system works. In 4 months of cutting way back on her sugar intake, she lost 15 pounds.

She has also found that she has more energy and that her sugar cravings are diminished. Not gone entirely, however. "I still crave it," she says. But when she does give in—when the devil on her shoulder is too loud to ignore—she is able to satisfy the craving with less sugar than she used to require.

It started during Lent in 2001, when Carrie decided to give up chocolate chip cookies. Her fiancé, John, joined her as a show of support. By the time Lent was over, she realized that cookies weren't calling to her as loudly as they had before.

"At first, that was a really big sacrifice for me," she says. "John and I used to make cookies every couple of weeks, during the winter holidays. I have always had a big sweet tooth, and he has, too. He doesn't have to watch his weight like I do, so it's hard. But now I find that one or two small cookies will do the trick instead of four or five. And that's fine with me."

Carrie is pleased with the changes she has made. She is eating a lot more fruit, and she and John have replaced their after-dinner cookies with sorbet and all-fruit ice pops. But she still finds that evenings, in front of the television, are difficult times to get through. It is then that she turns to her magazines or goes upstairs—away from the television and the kitchen.

*W I N N I N G   A C T I O N*

**Occupy your mind to stifle thoughts of the sweet stuff.**
*So many times, we eat not because we are hungry but because the food is there and we're thinking about it. But if we get our minds focused on something else, we can no longer hear the calls and can avoid the temptation to eat. Distraction is the worst enemy of the devil on your shoulder, even if the devil turns out to be a Devil Dog.*

# *SHE COULDN'T EAT JUST ONE— SO NOW SHE EATS NONE*

Jane Srygley learned the hard way that limiting the amount of sugar she ate didn't solve her cravings. "I would tell myself that today I'm going to have only a couple of bites of sugar," she says. "For a while that worked, but then I would eat a little bit today, a little more tomorrow, and end up going to the 7-Eleven and buying Twinkies and Slurpees and going crazy."

She kept resetting her internal "sugar clock" to small amounts of sweets and then losing control—until she had a revelation in 1996. "I had decided I was going to have two pieces of candy that day," says Jane, 38, of Newark, New Jersey. "After one bite, I started thinking that I should have a bit more than that. This lightbulb went on—just that one bite of sugar had made me want more. I realized that something that could get into my brain and mess with my priorities was something I didn't need in my life.

"My family has a history of alcoholism," Jane continues. "I realized this has got to be what it's like to take one drink and not be able to stop." She didn't pick up anything sweet for 4 years.

Her relapse occurred while trying to lose weight on a low-carbohydrate diet. "The authors of the diet seemed to make sense when they said you could have a little bit of sugar, as in a moderate dessert after dinner, and go low-carb the rest of the day," she says. "Well, within a week, I was in front of the vending machine buying five things. It was insane. I gained 18 pounds in 3 weeks."

After learning her lesson, Jane went cold turkey again. She's in the process of gradually cutting out anything remotely sweet: maple syrup, honey, molasses, even artificial sweeteners. "They have a lesser effect on me," she says, "but they seem to prime me to want more." The only sweet foods she intends to keep eating are fresh fruits and diluted fruit juice.

Jane takes special care when eating out. "You have to ask about the preparation in restaurants and make sure they don't add sugars," she says. "I can't go near Chinese food because they use sugar in everything.

"As hard as it was to give up sugar, once you've done it, you realize how little you're missing," says this executive assistant and as-piring opera singer. "I'll be dining with somebody who's having the dessert and will drool over it for a couple of minutes. But then I re-alize I missed a few minutes of pleasure and *days* of pain and agony, so it's totally worth it."

## WINNING ACTION

**Go cold turkey.** Sometimes, drastic measures are the best. And if you're like some people, who need only a taste of sugar to go on a binge, cutting the sweet stuff out of your diet entirely may be the way to go. If a permanent change is too overwhelming to contemplate, one strategy might be to give up sweets but allow yourself any other foods you want until you realize that you can live without sugar. Then you can make adjustments until you're eating nutritiously. Remember, you're trading in sweets for a healthier, happier, saner life. You're worth the effort!

# Lift Your Mood
# without Food

# *SHE TRADED DOUGHNUTS FOR A BEAUTY PAGEANT CROWN*

Giorgina Pinedo was 22, a new bride, and just plain lonely when she moved from her native Venezuela to New Jersey in 1989. "It was really hard for me, getting used to another country. I didn't have any family here. I didn't speak the language at all. I took refuge in food," says Giorgina, now 35. "I'd buy a dozen doughnuts every day and eat the whole box." If her husband (an airline pilot who was frequently away) had the car, Giorgina would hike 3 miles to the store rather than forfeit her daily sugar fix.

The 5-foot-2-inch, 115-pound beauty quickly put on weight. "I craved sugar constantly. I didn't want to give it up because it made me feel better. I always got a boost after I ate it," she says. In 1991, she and her husband moved to their present home in Orlando. By then, Giorgina had learned English, and she took a job at Walt Disney World. Even there, she munched on sweets all day long for comfort until, by 1995, she'd ballooned to 159 pounds.

"I was honestly miserable," remembers Giorgina. Desperate, she signed up at a nearby Jenny Craig weight-loss center in March 1996. Being required to eat only Jenny Craig foods "taught me portion control," says Giorgina. In 4 months, she shed 20 pounds. As she began to choose her own foods again, she worried about backsliding. But she didn't, and here's why.

While out shopping for new clothes, she struck up a conversation with a woman who was a beauty pageant judge. After hearing about Giorgina's recent weight loss, the woman recommended she enter the upcoming pageant, which was based largely on personal achievement. Giorgina said okay, and for the competition, she decided to share her story about her weight-loss success. She was dazzled when, weighing 139, she grabbed the title of Ms. Petite Orlando

1996. "That kept me motivated," she asserts. In fact, Giorgina had stumbled upon a well of inspiration.

Spurred on by the desire to win another beauty pageant, she kept on dieting. She learned to tackle cravings by eating fruit or carrots and to fend off anxiety by calling someone on the phone rather than reaching for a doughnut. In January 1997, she hired a personal trainer and began running 3 to 5 miles a day. "I put everything I had into it," she says. In 3½ months, she cast off 34 more pounds. She went on to win several more beauty contests and was crowned Ms. Florida U.S. Continental in 1999.

That same year, she earned a degree in nutrition and a personal trainer certification. She eventually landed her current job, hosting and producing fitness and nutrition shows and acting as assistant director of promotions for a Spanish language television station. She is also hostess, producer, and director of a very popular music show in Orlando. She's weighed about 105 pounds since 1997, and she's thrilled with her newfound beauty. "But it's not about how I look; it's about how I feel," she insists. "I am capable, confident, and no longer ashamed of myself."

### WINNING ACTION

**Set your sights on something worth quitting for.** *Giorgina's tale is all about motivation—beauty pageants provided her with a powerful source of inspiration. Follow her lead. Don't make giving up sweets your goal. Instead, let it be a step toward a greater end. Give yourself an objective—be it improved health, higher self-esteem, even a smaller dress size—and make a commitment to work at it every day.*

# *HE FINDS KNOWING THE ENEMY IS HALF THE BATTLE*

As an obstetrician, Asher B. Galloway of Douglasville, Georgia, often finds himself under stress and eating on the run. "You never know when someone's going to call you away from what you're doing," he says. "And when someone's in labor, you don't know how things will turn out. Tragedies are rare, but there's always the possibility of something going wrong."

Many times, Asher has to squeeze in his meals between patients—and that doesn't always lead to good choices. "We spend a lot of time at the hospital at night," he says—and with the hospital cafeteria closed, the only food available is the high-sugar variety from vending machines.

Things changed for Asher in early 1999, when he ran across the book *Sugar Busters!* and began educating himself about what sugar does to the body. "It's amazing," he says. "You don't realize how much sugar is in the regular American diet and how sweets can drag you down."

Even though Asher's field of work isn't nutrition, he was still able to do plenty of research on how sugar affects the body. "When your sugar level is consistently high, you need a chronically high level of insulin to deal with it," he says. "And scientists have observed that when your level of insulin increases, it drives up your cholesterol. It's known that people with diabetes tend to have a greater incidence of heart disease, coronaries, things like that.

"I'm convinced that the reason you shouldn't eat sugar is not to lose weight but to stay healthy," says Asher. "I've made the commitment to cut down on glucose (grape sugar), sucrose (table sugar), and maltose, which is in beer. I happen to like beer, but in the past couple of years, I've had only one."

Asher, who's 55, has also made a strong effort to stay away from the vending machines at the hospital, bringing in fruit to snack on and drinking sugar-free soda or merely steeling himself against the desire for sweets and carrying on with his work. "You have to be disciplined to stay away from that stuff," he says.

Asher's discipline has helped him drop 50 pounds, bringing him down to 250 on his 5-foot-10 frame. "Once I kept my blood sugar at a more constant level, it seemed that my metabolism worked more steadily and I felt better—like a natural high, I guess," he says. "I had more energy and seemed to be clearer in my mind."

### WINNING ACTION

**Learn what sugar does to your body.** *Even without a medical background, you can still find plenty of material on how sugar affects you in both the short term and over time. Reading this book is a good first step, and you can continue your education by speaking with nutritionists, reading medical journals and textbooks at college libraries, and visiting diabetes support groups to learn about their experiences. Being aware of what's happening inside your body can help curb impulses, even in the face of stress, and keep you running strong.*

## SHE PUT HER CRAVINGS ON HOLD

Tina Van Erp lived and worked in Germany for 3 years. While she was there, a very unusual thing happened. "I lost 15 pounds without even thinking about it," she says. "It didn't occur to me what was going on."

She would visit the United States every so often and be surprised by how "syrupy" everything tasted—but she didn't think more of it. Not, that is, until she moved back to Minneapolis for good in 1997 and constantly felt sick. "Everything I ate made me feel bad, and I gained weight without realizing it," she says.

Tina eventually determined that her weight gain and illness stemmed from the same source. "The difference in the amount of sugar in the food here put me in a whirlwind," she says. "Weight gain, the inability to lose weight or manage cravings through exercise, moodiness, general edginess—all came from the amount of sugar in the food."

Her first step in finding a solution to excessive sugar consumption was "to realize that my craving is a reaction to boredom or stress," she says, with boredom at work often being the cause of the stress. Sugary snacks, even though they tend to only worsen her anxiousness, serve as something emotionally distracting.

With this realization, Tina decided in 1999 to take a new approach to her snacking. "If I think a snack would be good, I tell myself I'll wait 10 minutes first," she says, "and if I still want it in 10 minutes, fine, I'll have it."

All too often, though, the phone rings or a coworker approaches her about a project. By the time she thinks about the snack again, a half hour has passed, and the craving has long since vanished.

In addition to delaying her snacks, Tina has tried to duplicate Europe's low-sugar foods by buying nothing with more than 3 grams of sugar per serving. "I don't eat most of what's in the grocery store," she says. "There's only one applesauce that's just apples and water, and most mainstream brands of peanut butter have loads of sugar in them." Tina prefers to shop in natural food stores, which have a better selection of low-sugar staples.

So far, these new habits have served this 34-year-old well. Says Tina, who is 5 feet 8 inches tall, "Staying away from sugar has decreased my mood swings and anxiety level throughout the day. It has also allowed my body to lose 10 pounds naturally and at its own speed."

### WINNING ACTION

**Wait 10 minutes before getting yourself a snack.** *But don't spend that time dreaming about how good the ice cream will taste when you finally get to it. Do something active instead, whether it's making a phone call, writing an e-mail message, or doing something around the house like vacuuming or loading the washer. The key is to get your mind on something other than eating. Your craving will often fade away and leave you wondering why you wanted something sweet in the first place.*

## SHE LEARNED TO POSTPONE HER INDULGENCES

Years ago, whenever Ann von Linden stressed out at work, she would plow through so many peanut M&M's that she'd wind up feeling sick. But these days, she waits until as late as possible in the workday to savor a few M&M's. "It gives me something to look forward to," she says. "And sometimes, if I wait long enough, it will be time for me to go home."

Ann, who's 40 and lives in Albany, New York, was always a big fan of sugar. Butterfinger candy bars, ice cream, and M&M's were among her favorites. Then in the late 1980s, while working at a group home for the disabled, she became super stressed. "I had a lot of long hours, and I was involved in the direct care of the residents," she says. "I was eating so many M&M's that I'd be nausated."

Around the same time, Ann decided to become a vegetarian and started shopping at a food co-op. She also picked up the book *Sugar Blues* and began to rethink the way she ate sweets. She realized that she was typically turning to sugar out of boredom and stress and that the white stuff was sending her body on crazy ups and downs that ultimately left her drained of energy.

Getting pregnant gave Ann even more incentive to stop eating sugar. But after her daughter was born in 1997, she couldn't stay away from sweets. Three years later, she got pregnant again. After her second daughter was born, Ann found sugar creeping back into her life—but this time, she seized control by trying healthier treats, cutting back on portions, and limiting indulgences to certain times of the day.

Now, every night after the kids are in bed, she helps herself to a half-cup of nondairy ice cream. She eats cookies sweetened with honey, maple syrup, or other natural sugars. She even allows herself a slice of cake during an occasional outing.

And during the day, she restricts M&M's to her office, where she is now the supervisor of a supportive apartment program, a job that involves less stress.

"I don't bring the M&M's home, and I don't eat them more often than every other day," she says. "When I do, I always try to wait until the end of the day. Sometimes, I eat none, and I go home saying, 'Another day without M&M's.' It makes me feel really good that I can control what I eat instead of letting food control me." In fact, sometimes Ann is so exhilarated by her restraint that she winds up eating no M&M's at all for several days, if not weeks.

*W I N N I N G   A C T I O N*

**Postpone your special treat to the end of your workday.**
*By saving sweets for later, you give yourself something to
look forward to. Perhaps by then, you'll be ready to head
home, and you may decide to skip indulging altogether.
Also, try limiting your treats to the work setting. They'll
be out of reach in the evenings and on weekends, when
you may be more apt to nibble.*

# SHE COOKS VEGETABLES BY THE POTFUL TO STAVE OFF BINGES

Growing up at the end of the Depression, Bobbi Falco took comfort
in sweets. When she was a young child, her mother baked a cake for
the family once a week. "It was always a big deal," recalls Bobbi, now
66 and a retired kindergarten teacher living in Aptos, California.
"Sugar had an unhealthy power over us. There was never any leftover cake at our house."

As a teen, Bobbi began bingeing and wrestling with bulimia. "I
was just driven to eat," she says. "I would buy a dozen doughnuts
and probably go through most of them. Then I would throw up and
eat ice cream or cake." After high school, Bobbi's tendency toward
bulimia subsided. But she struggled with bingeing—and weight
problems—throughout her life. Her highest weight, in 1976, was
210 pounds. She managed to lose some of that, but in 1998, she still
carried 205 pounds on her 5-foot-8 frame.

"I was desperate all my life on this issue," she admits. "I knew I
had a problem. I was not in control around food." Then, in February 1999, Bobbi became involved in an Internet site for sugar ad-

dicts, where she found the support she needed to change.

"I began buying lots of fresh vegetables, learning to cook them in tasty ways," she says. "Including a protein source with every meal and snack has been the most important component for me." Planning ahead, including getting the shopping done and having healthy food ready, is also very important, Bobbi explains. "If you forget to go shopping or wait too long between meals, you're more inclined to eat what you shouldn't."

These days, a typical dinner might include chicken or beef, brown rice, and vegetables such as broccoli or green beans cooked in chicken stock and seasoned with hot pepper flakes or garlic powder. She'll toss together a large salad with no dressing or steam two heads of cauliflower and season them with curry powder.

Whatever she and her husband don't eat that day, they save. "That way, when I open the fridge, I can see lots of good things," says Bobbi. "If I avoid sugar, I stay stable. If I have one cupcake, I want five." Vegetables, meats, oatmeal, and cottage cheese are all central to her diet now. She keeps sweet fruits to a minimum, since those, too, can set off cravings.

Since early 2000, Bobbi has lost about a half pound a week on her diet, which limits carbohydrates and gets 30 percent of calories from protein. Today, she weighs 180 pounds—only 10 pounds from her target weight of 170.

### WINNING ACTION

***Prepare healthy foods ahead of time.*** *Do you reach for the cookies whenever you're hungry, tired, or too busy to cook? Make a point of fixing yourself a mammoth salad (without dressing; add dressing at serving time so the greens don't wilt in the interim) or a potful of vegeta-*

*bles on the weekend—enough to last several days. That way, when you need a quick meal or snack at the end of a busy day, all you have to do is pull ready-made food from the fridge.*

## ONCE FULFILLED, SHE QUIT FILLING UP ON SWEETS

For 6 years, Alisa Bauman loved to snack on sweets while she was at work. Not anymore. Alisa quit her job and started her own freelance business in January 2001. She quickly discovered she'd left her cravings behind. "I think the cravings were the result of procrastination and unfulfillment," says Alisa, a 30-year-old writer from Emmaus, Pennsylvania. "I wasn't happy doing what I was doing."

Alisa remembers the first week she began working as a writer for a book publisher, back in 1994. After receiving negative feedback from her boss, she headed to a nearby bakery and bought two dozen cookies. She ate many of them. She wasn't really a binge eater, but she sought solace in sweets whenever she was under stress. Pretty soon, she was heading to the cafeteria nearly every day for a chocolate chip cookie or some other dessert. And when a coworker brought in baked goods, Alisa inevitably helped herself to one. And then another. And another. "If there was something sweet near me, all I could think about was the food," confesses Alisa. "I believe it was really tied in to the stress."

An active runner who exercised daily, 5-foot-3 Alisa kept her weight down to about 125 pounds. But every winter, she would gain a few pounds, then work hard to lose them. "If I kept this up, it was going to get ugly," she says.

Leaving her job helped her conquer her cravings in several ways. First and foremost, she no longer faces the daily stress induced by tasks she dreads. Once that stress disappeared, she felt more in control and took charge of her eating habits. She now keeps plenty of healthy snacks, like baby carrots, on hand and munches on them throughout the day.

Alisa makes it clear that she still has some work-related stress; she just no longer feels compelled to snack as a result of it. Instead, she heads outside and takes a walk, plays with her dog, or just sits for a while in the sun. When she gets back indoors, she's usually refreshed and ready to take on whatever job is waiting. "Before, I felt if I left my desk and went for a walk, people would look down on that," she explains.

When Alisa started her own business, a former coworker joked that she was bound to get fat working from home. In fact, in 3 months' time, Alisa's career change helped her drop from a high of 128 pounds to 121.

### WINNING ACTION

**Take control of your stress.** *Maybe you can't quit your job and start your own business. But if chocolate chip cookie cravings are ruling the day, it's probably a sign that you need to take charge of your situation. Ask yourself what solutions you can find to relieve your own stressful predicament. It could be as simple as taking a walk in the middle of the day. Think that would be frowned upon? Explain to your boss why you need it. In addition to helping put a lid on cravings, the short exercise break can refresh your mind so you're better able to handle your job.*

# SHE RAISED HER ENDORPHINS AND LOWERED HER SUGAR INTAKE

Kate McMurry has some very sweet childhood memories. "My mother was a home economics teacher," recalls the 50-year-old resident of Alexandria, Virginia. "She made fabulous chocolate chip cookies, snickerdoodles, chocolate cream pie, every kind of fabulous goodie you can imagine."

But Kate, a former therapist and now a freelance writer, recognized early on that her family tree was laden with relatives who suffered from diabetes, obesity, and heart disease. "Almost everybody in my lineage is thin when they're young but puts on weight beginning in their thirties," she explains. "Many weigh 200 pounds or more by age 35, and some get diabetes as a result of their obesity. I've tried everything to be different."

Though she's fought sugar cravings for most of her life, she's remained slim at 5 feet 7 inches and 132 pounds. She believes her commitment to exercise is one reason she's managed to outsmart her genetic tendency toward obesity. "The thing that's going to get you into sugar cravings is that you're not controlling your life," she asserts. "You're trying to alter your mood, and you turn to comfort food because it's a quick fix." Kate tries to keep her moods stable without treats.

To that end, she works out every day, as she has for many years. She feels that daily exercise boosts her mood and prevents her from growing dependent on sweets, because it raises her endorphins—chemicals produced in the brain that naturally reduce stress, depression, and anxiety. "If I see myself getting cravings, I know it's coming from an emotional vacuum," Kate says.

"My personal theory is that you should look for things that raise endorphins and are not destructive," she adds. Laughter and exercise both fit that bill. That's why Kate often works out in front of the TV. "I watch comedies that I have taped or videos of funny movies while I exercise, doubly raising my endorphins," she says.

Kate considers a 2-hour walk in a nearby park her optimum workout. Often, though, her schedule or the weather won't permit that. So instead, she rides her exercise bike, or she lays out a padded foam mat in front of the TV and walks in place. Either way, she's sure to get 30 to 50 minutes of exercise a day.

In 2000, Kate decided to try to lose 7 pounds and gave up sugar altogether. Again, exercise helped her achieve her goal. She discovered that if she chose to work out when she had a sugar craving, the craving evaporated. Kate lost those 7 pounds, and she has stayed around her present weight ever since.

### WINNING ACTION

**Exercise to raise your endorphins.** Is anxiety driving you to the candy aisle? Drive to the gym instead. Regular aerobic exercise can stimulate the release of mood-lifting endorphins that help you fight cravings. If you want to bump up your endorphins, keep in mind that the duration of the exercise is more important than intensity. So choose a low-impact aerobic activity, like walking, biking, or swimming, and do it five or six times a week for 30 to 45 minutes at a stretch.

## HE CHOSE STRETCHING OVER SWEETS

Howard Mickel abused sugar for most of his life. First as a young Ph.D. candidate and then throughout his 22-year academic career,

Howard binged on sugar whenever he faced tight deadlines or complex writing projects. "I would sit down with my work and a carton of six colas and a box of cookies, and most of it would be gone by evening's end," confides the retired philosophy professor, who's now 76 and living in La Jolla, California. "The tension would be worked off through junk food."

Even after he retired in 1987, he gorged on junk food daily. Every morning after breakfast, he'd drive to a 7-Eleven to pick up a croissant with powdered sugar, two chocolate cupcakes with cream filling, and a 32-ounce cola—a habit he'd kept up since about 1970. A former competitive runner and racewalker (he still walks 2 miles a day), Howard's active lifestyle enabled him to avoid obesity.

Nevertheless, in 1990, he was 15 pounds overweight. "One day, I got distressed looking at my tummy in store windows as I walked past," he says. He knew if he wanted to shed some pounds, he'd have to shake off his sugarcoated eating habits.

So he did. He traded his cola for a less sugary iced tea and began eating more fruits and vegetables so hunger wouldn't drive him to junk food. Over several months, he lost the 15 extra pounds, bringing him to his present weight of 175 at 6 feet 1 inch tall. Even under stress, he downed notably less sugar. But Howard, who still writes for academic journals, continued to turn to sweets whenever a deadline loomed.

In 1996, he took a class in yoga to help him better manage stress. Now, yoga and other relaxation methods have replaced his once-desperate need for sugar. For 3 years, he participated in a weekly yoga class. Then, in 1999, after being diagnosed with Parkinson's disease, Howard started practicing yoga daily. He now begins every morning with a 40-minute yoga routine. He follows that with 20 minutes of progressive relaxation—relaxing his entire body slowly, beginning with the toes and working upward. Those exercises keep his body flexible and make stress reduction a daily experience for him.

He no longer faces the rigid deadlines of academia, but his Parkinson's disease has brought him many frustrations. "Now, it takes me three or four times the effort to type something," he points out. When tensions rise, he sometimes relies upon deep-breathing exercises to relax himself.

Howard allows himself one candy bar after lunch every day and one 8- to 12-ounce glass of soda with a meal five times a week. But he doesn't binge anymore. "Now, I do yoga," he says.

### WINNING ACTION

**Take up yoga.** *Do you rely on sugar binges to get you through times of high stress? Yoga and its counterparts deep breathing and progressive relaxation are all proven stress busters. The deep stretches performed during a yoga routine simultaneously tone the body and relax the mind. Yoga positions are most effective when done consistently, and they are best learned from an instructor. Check adult education programs, gyms, and other health-oriented institutions to find a class near you.*

## SHE PUT HER SNACK HABIT TO BED

Grace Penny knows that overeating is often unrelated to appetite. "Boredom," she says, "leads to mindless picking at foods." That's why this 65-year-old retired special education teacher from Lutz, Florida, thinks carefully before giving in to a craving. What she's learned is that she's better off hitting the sack than having a snack.

In 1998, Grace, measuring only slightly more than 5 feet, weighed 205 pounds. She'd been carrying that extra weight for 35 years and often indulged in sweets thoughtlessly. "At work, we had a regular supply of homemade frosted apple-cinnamon buns and coffee with whole milk and sugar," she says. What's more, Grace loved rich desserts like cheesecake and often treated herself to after-dinner sweets.

Such habits took their toll. In 1996, Grace was diagnosed with type 2 diabetes and high cholesterol. "I was beginning to feel unwell all the time," she explains. "My heartbeat seemed loud, I wasn't sleeping well, and I was aware that my daughter and husband were very concerned." Her health worries prompted her, in May 1998, to sign up for a monthlong stay at Duke University's Rice Diet Program in Durham, North Carolina.

The program introduced her to daily exercise, along with a high-fiber, low-salt, low-fat diet built around fresh fruits, grains, and vegetables. Instructors taught her a number of strategies for maintaining her diet. One that Grace has found helpful is to think carefully before giving in to a craving.

"I try to apply the acronym HALT: Am I *Hungry*? *Angry*? *Lonely*? *Tired*?" she says. More often than not, she isn't hungry at all.

"According to the Duke nutritionists, people confuse tiredness and hunger more than any other sensations. That was true for me," Grace explains. "I've learned that when a craving hits really hard, I have mixed up *hungry* with *tired*, and I go to bed."

If the craving hits midday, she takes a catnap. When she finds herself yearning for sweets at night, she calls it a day. "Rarely do I wake up and even remember the craving feeling!" she insists.

If Grace can't nap, she boosts her energy with a brisk walk. She also seeks to keep her energy high through daily exercise—a minimum of 1 hour of water aerobics a day.

Grace went off her cholesterol and diabetes medications within a week of joining the Duke program and has managed to maintain healthy glucose and cholesterol levels without drugs since that time. She lost 50 pounds in 7 months and dropped another 10 pounds over time, bringing her to her present weight of 145, closer to her ultimate goal of 115.

### WINNING ACTION

**Go to bed when fatigue-induced cravings strike.** *A 20-minute power nap can be your best energy booster. Unlike sugar, which gives you a brief surge, a nap energizes you for the rest of the day. So if you regularly find yourself reaching for a candy bar in the late afternoon or a brownie right before bed, it may be fatigue that's fueling your unhealthy habit. Give your body what it really needs—a soothing rest.*

## A JOURNAL KEPT HER HONEST WHEN SHE QUIT SUGAR COLD TURKEY

Ever since her college days, Tracey Kaufman has used a journal to help her survive broken romances. So when it came time to end her love affair with sugar, Tracey once again turned to journaling for support.

Tracey, who's 37 and lives in San Bruno, California, was a self-described sugar addict who loved ice cream and anything chocolate. "I was such a chocoholic and sugar addict that if I ate it, I'd need more," she says. "Every day at 3:00, I'd need a sugar fix. And during the holidays, my hand would always be in the candy bowls."

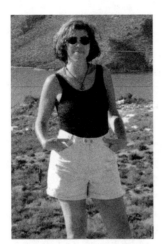

Writing in a journal helped Tracey discover why she loved sweets.

For years, Tracey suffered from fatigue. Her winter colds started up in November and didn't quit until May. She also had stomach pains, headaches, and acne. Then she read *The Macrobiotic Way: The Complete Macrobiotic Diet & Exercise Book*, which suggested that her symptoms might be linked to her diet.

The book revolutionized her thinking. On her 34th birthday, she went out to dinner and finished the meal with a chocolate shake. The next day, she stopped eating sugar cold turkey. She also saw an alternative health nutritionist who analyzed her symptoms and told her she was lactose intolerant. She was advised to give up all animal proteins, dairy foods, and artificial sweeteners.

Tracey started eating more miso, tempeh, and soy products so she could avoid foods she couldn't tolerate while still getting plenty of nutrients. She gave up alcohol and avoided all refined sugars and sweeteners. And every night, at the end of a sugar-free day, she'd remind herself of her goals in her journal.

"I also made lists of things I'd stay away from and wrote down the triggers that set me off," she says. "Then I made lists of things I could do instead of eating sugar, such as taking a bath, shopping, or going to the movies."

Writing in a journal every night helped keep her honest and faithful to her goals. "If I ever cheated, I'd have to lie to myself," she says. "And you just can't lie when you write in a journal."

The nightly writings also helped her realize that her sugar cravings were driven by emotion. She wanted sugar when she felt depressed, lonely, and unappreciated but also when she was celebrating and in the mood to treat herself. "I never ate sugar out of hunger," she says.

It took Tracey 3 months to tame her cravings, but her health improved within a month. Her headaches disappeared, her energy levels improved, and her complexion cleared up. And she almost never gets colds anymore. As an unexpected bonus, she shed 17 pounds from her 5-foot-5 frame and weighed just 120 after 8 months without sugar. Some of the weight has come back since then as the result of a lack of exercise, Tracey says.

Tracey has resumed eating fish and drinks an occasional glass of wine. She satisfies her rare cravings by eating fruit or desserts made with sweeteners like brown rice syrup, stevia, and honey.

Writing in her journal helped Tracey survive the tough early months of life without sugar. But once she stopped eating it, she found she no longer craved it. "You just need a good enough reason," she says. "And for me, it was my health."

## WINNING ACTION

**Keep a journal when you decide to cut back on sugar.**
*Jotting down the reasons you want to quit will help you stay focused on your goals. It may also help you uncover the reasons you crave sweets and alleviate some of your stress. Research has shown that expressive writing can help improve the immune system and ease pain. Journaling is also widely touted by programs such as Weight Watchers as a tool to help promote weight loss.*

# *SHE TALKS HERSELF OUT OF SUGAR*

Renee Palmer thought she was doing herself a favor when she indulged in fat-free sweets. But when she discovered how much sugar they contained, she decided to ditch the sweets and rely on positive self-talk to keep herself focused.

Renee was always surrounded by sugar. Her grandmother worked in a candy factory, her grandfather for an ice cream company. She's spent most of her life on a yo-yo diet and has always tried to steer clear of high-fat foods. "I'd convinced myself that if it was fat-free, it was okay," says Renee, who's 35 and lives in Burlington, North Carolina. "So then I was eating a fat-free, high-sugar diet."

Her weight problems didn't impede her love of running, and in January 2000, Renee ran her first marathon. But when her job as a speech-language pathologist became more stressful and her husband began traveling a lot for his work, Renee became lonely and depressed. She ate more sweets, stopped running, and started gaining weight. "When you start putting on weight, that just sets off another emotional trigger, and you eat more," she says.

By October 2000, her weight had peaked at 200 pounds, well above what's considered healthy for her 5-foot-6 frame. She was short of breath, her feet ached, and she suffered from acid reflux. On Halloween, at her doctor's urging, Renee decided to quit sugar cold turkey and adopt the *Sugar Busters!* eating plan. Protein helped keep sugar cravings in check most of the time, as did a more healthy choice of snacks such as fruits, vegetables, and nuts.

The temptation grew stronger during the holidays, when the office was loaded with sweets. "The mental game set in when

I saw Christmas candy in the break room at work," she says. "I would tell myself to think of it as a helping of poison, because it had virtually the same effect on me. It was killing me slowly."

She also began repeating mantras to help her stay on course. "I engaged in positive self-talk and mini-mantras such as 'You are strong' or 'If you eat that, it will only make you feel bad,'" she says. "This was the most helpful thing I could do for myself when I felt the weakest, and it worked."

It helped that Renee found a new, less stressful job and that her husband eventually got a job requiring less travel. She has also learned to tell her colleagues up front that she no longer eats sugar. "Now, I just say, 'I can't have that,'" she says. "If they ask why, I just say that I don't eat refined sugar and white flour."

Renee's positive self-talk has paid off, and she now weighs 150 pounds. She continues to stay away from candy and does a new self-talk that focuses on her next goal: to run a second marathon. "I tell myself, 'Athletes don't put junk into their bodies,'" she says. "If I can run a marathon, then I am an athlete, and I should adopt that mind-set. If I put junk into my body, then I will get junk out of it. The self-talk helps me to evaluate something before I eat it mindlessly and regret it later."

### WINNING ACTION

**Talk yourself out of eating sugar.** *Remind yourself of your goal and why you are trying to avoid sugar. Whether you are striving for athletic achievement, trying to lose weight, or simply needing a reminder that sugar is no good, a little positive self-talk may be all it takes for you to avoid that candy bar. Repeat your mes-*

*sage a few times and you may find that your craving has passed.*

## *SHE TRAINED HER BRAIN TO AVOID SUGAR*

As a registered nurse in Sarasota, Florida, Elizabeth Bohorquez never had much time to think about what she was eating. "Nurses tend to have bad dietary habits, and I was no different," she says. "I helped myself to what I wanted when I wanted it. Certainly, I was a 'walk-by' eater and never said no when the offerings appealed to my eyes.

"I can remember eating even when my stomach ached. If I woke in the middle of the night, a cookie accompanied me back to bed," says Elizabeth.

"After my children were born, I started to 'pay the piper,' but I never connected my health problems to my sugar addiction," she continues. "My emotions ran high, my fatigue had become chronic, and my weight yo-yoed dramatically," reaching a peak of 180 pounds in her late forties. "I was better if I exercised, but as the years progressed, the hunger became insatiable."

Although she thought she had a healthy diet, Elizabeth examined her food choices more closely. "I came to understand how they were related to my family's medical history, as well as my own," she says. "I had been on every sort of diet imaginable throughout the years, but I had never understood how and why my body needed what it did."

Now she could see that her own sugar addiction had long roots in her family tree. It revealed a physical imbalance that, left unchecked, could lead to serious illness—heart disease, cancer, and diabetes. Wanting to avoid these conditions, Elizabeth vowed to get her sugar cravings under control.

Drawing on her decades of experience in the field of medical hypnosis, Elizabeth used self-hypnosis to increase her awareness of her cravings and to change her responses to them. "I became my most important patient," she says. "Since this was a lifestyle change, I had to design a program that would meet all my physical needs, as well as work out how I would manage those foods I did really enjoy."

She also trained in mental biofeedback, a relaxation technique that changes her physiological state to relieve cravings. "I have a higher level of communication with my body," says Elizabeth.

Next, she had to address the emotions as well as all the compulsive behaviors that go along with addiction. "As I learned to identify the emotions connected with my food issues, I was able to influence them with interactive self-hypnosis techniques I had designed for my cancer patients," Elizabeth explains. "With these tools, you feel a sense of power over your body and mind."

Elizabeth, now 61, stresses that each person's war against sugar addiction never ends. Someone can never say she is cured, because that person's physiology creates a tendency toward this behavior. "Managing sugar addiction is not a part-time job," she says. "Each day, I wake up and begin again."

Difficult as it may be, Elizabeth has succeeded well since she found her cure. When she began her program, she carried 185 pounds on her 5-foot-4 frame. Today, she maintains her weight at 130. "More than a decade has passed," she says, "and I'm healthier than ever before!"

*WINNING ACTION*

**Use self-hypnosis to quell your sugar desires.** *Through self-hypnosis, you can gain a deeper understanding of the relationship between your mind and your body—and its role in your cravings for sweets. You can also change your response to cravings, so they don't seem so overpowering. Your doctor or your local hospital should be able to refer you to a qualified health professional who can provide basic training in self-hypnosis techniques. The brain rules the body, so learn how to use it to its fullest.*

# SETTING ATHLETIC GOALS HELPED HER AVOID ENERGY-SAPPING SWEETS

In her youth, Teri Currie easily got away with eating Ring Dings for dinner. But when she got older and realized that sugar hindered her performance as a runner, Teri knew she had to ditch the sugar if she wanted to improve her times.

Teri, 38, of Albany, New York, grew up eating a lot of sweets. Her mother often used cookies to soothe unhappy feelings. "If I didn't eat dinner because there was spinach on my plate, she'd send me to bed," Teri recalls. "But then she'd come in later with Oreos because she felt sorry and wanted to make sure I knew she loved me."

In high school, Teri was an athlete who rarely ate dinner at home and instead gorged on Ring Dings and Devil Dogs for sustenance. In college, she ate lots of ice cream and cookies because they were inexpensive and accessible. Looking back, she realizes the sweets also helped make her feel better. "Sugar always made me happy for the moment," she says. "Whenever I felt clueless and lonely, sugar helped fill a void."

Then at 21, Teri discovered she had diabetes, and nurses and doctors warned her against sugar. But it wasn't until 3 years later, when she was hospitalized, that Teri knew she had to change her ways. "I couldn't breathe, and I couldn't urinate," she says. "It really scared me."

Teri started eating more fruits, vegetables, and grains. Eventually, she became a vegetarian. "But I continued to eat a lot of sugar—maybe because I was in denial," she says.

She also started running competitively in local races. She soon realized that she didn't have the stamina she had in her youth.

Making good time on her runs became important to Teri and gave her the impetus to limit her sugar intake. And sure enough, her times got better when she stopped eating sugar. So did her weight: She dropped 10 pounds from her 5-foot-8 frame, and she's still holding steady at 145.

But it's the improvement in her running that has pleased Teri most. A 3½-mile run that used to last as long as 35 minutes now takes as little as 26 minutes. "If you eat sugar, it just doesn't take you very far," she says. "You don't have any endurance, and you burn it off quickly. So I tell myself, 'If you eat this, your time is going to be really bad.' Now, I eat a banana before I run."

Teri continues to run 3½ miles every day, and she still competes in local races. She has also been successful at restricting her sugar intake to an occasional cookie, and she fights off cravings with sugar-free chewing gum. "I can definitely control it now," she says.

*WINNING ACTION*

**Take up a sport or other activity that requires you to perform at your peak, then set goals for it.** *Whether it's running a good time, winning a number of tennis matches, or swimming a certain distance, fitness goals give you added inspiration and incentive to ditch the sweets. And if you indulge during training while you're working toward your goal, you'll quickly learn why they call sugar empty calories. It tends to give you a surge of energy, then leave you sluggish and tired, hardly the condition that will help you reach your athletic goals.*

# RAISINS ARE HER SWEET SUBSTITUTE FOR DESSERT

Annie Grogan has fallen in love with raisins. And for good reason. They have helped her win the battle against desserts, a victory that has improved her life significantly.

"Raisins are awesome!" says Annie. "They are so sweet they satisfy my sweet tooth."

Annie, who's 29 and lives in Bozeman, Montana, describes herself as a sugar junkie. "Breakfast, lunch, and dinner—I was always eating a dessert," she says. "A cinnamon roll for breakfast, ice cream for lunch, and snacks all the time. It was pretty bad."

So bad that on New Year's Day 2001, she resolved to eliminate sweets from her diet. "I had a friend who was lifting weights, and she had gone almost a year without sugar," she says. "I thought it would be interesting to try. And boy, has it ever!"

Within a month, Annie started feeling better. "Sugar made me a little emotionally disturbed, unstable, unsure of myself," she says. "Now, I am definitely a lot clearer in my thoughts. I feel a lot more confident and have higher self-esteem. I can't prove that has anything to do with the sugar, but I have noticed it since I cut back on sweets."

Annie says she also has more energy and is able to sleep better. "I thought I felt good before," she says. "But compared with now, I was very lethargic."

Annie says the simple fact that she feels so much better is incentive enough to stay away from the cookie jar. But at the start of her diet, she struggled to resist the desserts to which she was accustomed. That's where the raisins came in—raisin bagels, in particular, were very satisfying when a sugar craving hit.

"I would put a little peanut butter on them or maybe a sliced banana," she says. "It is amazing how quickly foods develop a real sweetness. When I don't eat as much sugar, I taste flavors better."

Annie is convinced that she will be able to stick to her diet. And she has a piece of advice for those interested in following her example: "Don't substitute things that are bad for you for sugar. I thought since I wasn't eating as much sugar, I could eat a whole bag of potato chips. That wasn't a good idea."

### W I N N I N G   A C T I O N

**Grab a raisin bagel when a sugar craving hits.** *The raisins are sweet, and the bagel is high in carbohydrates, providing plenty of energy and not much fat (as long as you skip the butter or cream cheese). Make the bagel a whole grain one, and get plenty of vitamins, minerals, fiber, and good-for-you phytochemicals in the bargain. And if a bagel isn't handy,* *a small handful of raisins may be the key to appeasing your sugar craving without getting all the fat and calories that cakes, cookies, and candy bars carry with them.*

## *SHE TRADED CHOCOLATE FOR WATER*

For Donna Gerhart, sugar and work once went hand in hand. Coworkers doled out doughnuts at least one morning a week. Holidays and birthdays merited an in-house celebration for which Donna, a 48-year-old inventory control clerk from Allentown, Pennsylvania, benevolently baked a cake (chocolate with peanut butter icing was her favorite). Snacking on candy bars was often a group experience. "If somebody here was stressed out and had a candy bar, we'd all have one," says Donna.

Donna's penchant for treats didn't end when she left work for the day. At home, she typically downed a bowl of ice cream before bed—a nightly snack habit carried over from her childhood.

All those sweets took their toll. By 1998, Donna, who is 5 feet 3 inches, weighed 206 pounds. In January 1999, after her doctor recommended she lose weight to lower her cholesterol, she joined Weight Watchers. She immediately heeded her instructor's advice and began substituting water for snacks. "I can count on one hand the number of candy bars I've eaten since that time," she says.

Willpower alone impelled her to take some important steps, like packing away her baking pans and leaving the ice cream at the grocery store. But this self-proclaimed chocoholic credits her increased consumption of water for enabling her to resist temptation at work. "When you're craving something, most times your body just needs to be hydrated," Donna says, quoting her Weight Watchers instructor.

Donna relies on a 20-ounce bottle to keep the water flowing throughout the day. Every morning, she fills that bottle before going to work. She drinks it, and halfway through the day, she refills it. At home, she has a water cooler filled with spring water. "I put my mug under every time I go by, and have a drink," Donna says. And before bed? She doesn't need a snack. "I don't eat anything after supper," she says. "I just drink water."

Donna estimates she drinks the equivalent of six to seven 8-ounce glasses of water every day. She also takes fruit to work. Bananas, kiwis, plums, whatever is in season, she stores in the office refrigerator. When her coworkers go off to have a candy bar or a doughnut, Donna munches on fruit and sips her water instead. If someone else brings in a cake (Donna rarely bakes anymore), she may have a small piece, then she returns to her fruit and water.

Drinking water has helped Donna wash away 46 pounds over a 2-year period. She now weighs 159 pounds and is only a few pounds away from her target weight of 155.

### WINNING ACTION

**Drink more water.** *Keeping your body hydrated has a number of health benefits. You need water to carry nutrients and oxygen to your cells and to remove toxins. Dehydration, on the other hand, can leave you feeling lethargic. If you habitually turn to sugar to boost your energy, try this different tack. You just may find your body needs more water. Eight 8-ounce glasses a day is the usual recommendation, but you may be able to satisfy your cravings on less.*

# *SINCE GIVING UP WINE, SHE NO LONGER WANTS SWEETS*

Roslyn Balmagia says that when she was growing up, she had no choice but to clean her plate. "I had to finish everything," she says. "I remember battles over food where I'd say I wasn't hungry. The response was, 'You can't go out and play if you don't eat.'"

Cookies and sweets were always in the house. "This resulted in my overeating," says Roslyn, 46, of Sherman Oaks, California. "The more anxious or nervous I got, the more food I piled on. There were always issues with food, food being both friend and foe."

In October 2000, though, Roslyn made an interesting discovery after fasting for Yom Kippur. "Fasting was more difficult than usual because I felt sick," she says. "Following the fast, I just looked at some wine and felt nauseous. I realized that I was probably drinking more wine than I should have been, so I switched to water instead. The water helped cleanse me.

"I had always enjoyed wine with a meal, thinking it was a good thing," Roslyn continues. "But when I let go of the wine, I let go of the cravings for sugar. I am so much more balanced now after discovering the magic of drinking more water."

Roslyn admits that it's not easy to eat well when cravings strike. But once she recognized that her cravings seemed to be related to alcohol, she found herself in a better state of mind with regard to food. "My preferences shifted to proteins, fruits, and veggies. I lost a lot of bloat and stabilized my weight when I changed my food choices."

She used to keep company with Ben & Jerry's frozen yogurt. "I don't have it anymore," says Roslyn. "And when I eat cookies with the kids, my body lets me know I shouldn't. I've found that the prospect of living longer is making me want to live better. I just need to listen to my body and heed the messages it sends me."

## W I N N I N G   A C T I O N

**Cut back on—or eliminate—alcohol.** *Alcoholic drinks, including wine, beer, and hard liquor, are the nutritional equivalent of water and fermented sugar. They contain calories and not much else. You might as well drink a regular, sugar-laden soda. So if you're trying to cut back on your sugar consumption, pay as much attention to what's in your glass as what's on your plate. To quench your thirst and refresh yourself, try ice water with a squeeze of lemon or lime juice, sugar-free flavored water, or unsweetened iced tea.*

# SHE FOUND THE STRENGTH ONLINE TO QUIT SUGAR

Debbie Nedelman used to rely on the Internet just to sell things and do research. But it's become a source of support and motivation as she steers clear of sugar and sticks with her new way of eating.

Debbie, 40, of Miami, was an emotional eater most of her life, with chocolate her sweet of choice. A visit from her ex-husband could send her into a sugar binge just as easily as a sappy wedding commercial on TV. During a sad movie, she could dig her way through a half-gallon of ice cream. "Sometimes, it was so bad that I'd eat something even if I didn't like it," she says. "I remember eating cookies I hated. It was like a drug. You don't care what kind you're eating, as long as you're getting that sugar."

After being overweight all her life and trying several diets, Debbie stumbled onto *Sugar Busters!* She read the book twice and made up her mind that she was going to succeed this time. But she didn't want to tell her family or friends that she was trying yet another diet. "They'd say, 'Oh yeah, right,'" she says.

Instead, she found support on the Internet, on a Web site called www.3fatchicks.com. Shortly after she first logged on, she was asked to moderate a message board devoted just to people following the *Sugar Busters!* recommendations. "I put all my energy and time into this, and it motivated me to stay on the plan," Debbie says. "It has definitely kept me in line. Being the moderator, I think the girls look up to me, so I feel obligated to be good."

Debbie found plenty of support from others just like her, women who desperately wanted to share their experiences. "Some people are in touch on a daily basis," she says. "I've had days when I've been on the message board 11 times."

She has personally met five women through the message board. "You get to care about these people," she says. "We help each other through the hard times and congratulate each other on our triumphs."

More than a year after she changed her way of eating, Debbie, who is 5 feet 1½ inches tall, had lost 65 pounds and weighed 129 pounds. She's maintaining that weight. She walks six mornings a week, 4½ miles a day, and continues to follow the *Sugar Busters!* plan.

Sentimental commercials, sad movies, and even her ex-husband no longer send her on a binge. Best of all, Debbie has tamed her chocolate cravings. "About a week and a half ago, I had a piece of chocolate, a quarter ounce," she says. "I was so scared that one little square would make me fly into a feeding frenzy. But it did not. To me, this is much more amazing than the weight loss, to finally say that chocolate doesn't have the hold on me it once had."

## SHE PLANTED VEGETABLES AND CANNED HER CRAVINGS

Juanita Hansen knows that a bad mood can set off a sugar craving. "When I was depressed, I grabbed for the candy," admits the 53-year-old homemaker from Aurora, Colorado. But since she began battling her cravings, she's learned a thing or two about giving in to a bad mood. Gardening, she's discovered, is far better for the soul than sweets.

"Out in the garden, there is always something to do, like pull weeds. That in itself is a stress reliever," she says. While she was raising her children in the 1970s, Juanita "had a garden the size of a city block!" she recalls. But moving to Colorado in 1983 and living in apartments for the next 12 years left her without a vegetable patch. Juanita admits she had a hard time controlling her sugar cravings during those years.

Then in 1995, she and her husband bought a house, which

meant she could dig in the garden once again. Juanita noticed that tending to plants calmed her nerves. "When I'd get angry or upset, I'd just grab the hoe and head out to the garden," she says. "I lost track of time out there, but I always felt better when I got done."

With gardening doing such wonders for her nerves, Juanita realized she could stay away from the sweets she had been craving before she headed outside. Still, she wasn't able to completely weed sugar from her diet.

That was particularly true in 2000, when she underwent surgery for breast cancer and received radiation treatments and chemotherapy for several months afterward. While she beat the cancer, her cravings returned with a vengeance. Even though she was able to resume gardening in the spring, "I didn't feel up to par," she says.

Then in January 2001, Juanita paid a routine visit to her chiropractor. After hearing about her sugar cravings, he told her that she probably had too-high levels of the yeast *Candida albicans* in her body. The yeast can cause sugar cravings, he explained—and eating too much sugar feeds the yeast.

Not all health professionals agree with the *C. albicans* diagnosis or with the theory that the yeast can spread throughout the body. But it rang true for Juanita. On her chiropractor's advice, she eliminated sugar from her diet and drank tea made from reishi mushrooms to combat the yeast. She also took acidophilus and L-glutamine supplements after reading that they can help control *C. albicans*.

Since starting this regimen, Juanita says her sugar cravings have diminished. Still, when she's depressed or stressed out, she longs for sweets.

Her chief weapon? Her 30-by-45-foot vegetable garden. When a craving hits, "I head out to the garden with a water bottle," she says. "If anything is ready for picking, like young carrots, strawberries, or even peas, I'll rinse them off well with the garden hose and munch a bit. Some things don't make it to the dinner table! But mainly, I just drink water to stay away from the sweets."

Of course, she can't garden during winter months, but she spends hours inside plotting the design and rotation of her plants. In early March, as soon as the ground is workable, she begins planting. "I'm out there as often as I can be," she says. "When you focus on the garden, it helps you get back in touch with the earth."

### W I N N I N G   A C T I O N

***Get into the garden.*** *When you face a difficult situation, don't let your diet go to seed. Instead, plant a garden. Tending even a small patch of vegetables or flowers can be pleasantly absorbing, at once soothing your mood and keeping your mind off sweets. If you don't have the space for a regular garden, do container gardening. Plant in large pots or window boxes that you can place on your deck, balcony, or patio. In the winter, spend quality time with seed catalogues planning the upcoming season. Or garden indoors under grow lights—at the very least, you can keep some culinary herbs thriving. Tending the plants gets you out of the kitchen and away from sugary temptations.*

## SHE VISUALIZES THE ILL EFFECTS OF SUGAR

At her weakest moments, Jenna Norwood finds herself fantasizing about Dairy Queen's chocolate-dipped ice cream cones.

"I try to ignore it," says Jenna, 35. "Sometimes, it is very hard to resist."

But Jenna has found a way to chase off the image and to stop its whispers in her ear. "Now I visualize how I feel if I eat something like that," she says. "I realize that the sugar is not worth it."

Jenna, who lives in Sarasota, Florida, owns a public relations company. Sugar binges that she used to indulge in, spurred by stress from her job, would send her on emotional roller-coaster rides. "My happiness level would fluctuate," she says. "Sugar has a numbing effect, like a tranquilizer. I was in a cloud, and I was not getting as much done as I should."

And to add to that, there was guilt. "I couldn't get enough sugar, but I felt so guilty eating it," she says. "It was a negative emotional effect and a negative physical effect."

Jenna first swore off sugar in 1998, after making the connection that it was causing her to have headaches. At the end of a complete year without ice cream and cookies, she permitted herself a celebration—featuring sweets.

"I thought I had it under control," she says. "But I got back into the whole sugar cycle again."

After periods on and off the wagon, she resolved again on New Year's Day 2001 to cut out the sweets. "I was absolutely determined that I would conquer it this time," she says. Four months after making that resolution, Jenna was sticking to it.

"I completely abstain now," she says. "If someone brings dessert to work, I know that I can't have even one bite. One bite and I always go back for more."

Jenna has lost 6 pounds—at 5 feet 6 inches, she weighs 136—and is working to lose about 10 more. But even without weight loss, the diet is well worth the effort, she says.

"My energy level is so much better," she says. "My headaches are gone. I have no guilt. I just feel happier."

## *WINNING ACTION*

***Keep fresh in your mind how sugar makes you feel.***
*Without that image, a slice of cake or piece of chocolate is just something to satisfy your hunger and please your taste buds. But vivid visualizations of low energy, mood swings, and depressing guilt can help you see that tasty treat for what it really is: the enemy in your battle against cravings. Then, even a chocolate-dipped ice cream cone has no power.*

# Sugar's Gone–And So Are the Pounds

# *A CHANGE OF HEART CURED HIS CRAVINGS*

For Jeffrey Maitles, the decision to cut his sugar intake and lose weight came in 1997, during a shocking moment of self-awareness. "I was commenting to someone how overweight he was and how he should do certain things about it," says Jeffrey, of Encino, California. "Then I realized I was in the same position. I woke up to the fact that if I'm so good at telling other people what to do, it's time to make the decision myself."

But that decision didn't require Jeffrey to adopt restrictive eating habits or a punitive exercise regimen. "I'm a total disbeliever in any form of diet," he says. "Weight loss has to be done slowly because otherwise, the pounds will come right back."

For Jeffrey, his biggest success came with a change of attitude and his approach toward food. "You don't have to eat less. You can actually eat more often, but only when you're hungry and only if you stop once you're full," he says. He eats as often as six to eight times per day, but some "meals" consist of only a mouthful or two. "You can still get the pleasure, but you don't have to suffer the consequences," he explains.

He also takes more time with each of those meals. "I was always a fast eater—5 minutes and it was gone," says Jeffrey. "Then I started to slowly chew my food, 20 or 30 times, and really appreciate and enjoy it."

Jeffrey also quit his habit of taking a swig of soda with every bite. "Every mouthful, I'd wash the food down," he says. "I cut out all the sodas and drink only water."

He even cut the treats that his wife always made for him—at his request. "I was always asking for desserts," says Jeffrey, "and my wife was a very good cook, making pies, apple crumbles, and bread puddings."

Two years of eating with a new attitude (and a small amount of weight lifting) brought Jeffrey's weight down from 205 to 165. After 2 more years, the 5-foot-11-inch 46-year-old saw his weight settle in at 175 pounds, and he doesn't expect that to change in the future.

"I always stress the importance of attitude," he says. "Even without dieting, if you stand in front of a mirror with your clothes off and tell yourself, 'Yes, you're looking good today,' you can place this thought in your mind to assist you in losing weight. And then you're going to be careful about what you consume."

### W I N N I N G   A C T I O N

**Think of cutting back on sweets as a change in lifestyle, not a diet.** *A diet implies a temporary change in eating habits to accomplish a particular goal. But if your goal is to reduce your sugar consumption permanently, you must also adjust your behavior permanently. Without a change in attitude, you'll go back to your old ways at the slightest provocation. But gradually incorporating new habits, like taking the time to chew slowly, can be as much of a boost as anything else and provide the impetus for staying sugar-free.*

## SHE QUIT SUGAR FOR 10 DAYS AND TURNED IT INTO A LIFETIME

In 1965, Jeri Jefferis decided to give up sugar for 10 days. Over 36 years later, she is still sugar-free. By telling herself that she was quitting sugar for only a short spell, Jeri was able to kick the sugar habit for good.

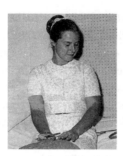

Thirty-six years after giving up sweets, Jeri feels and looks better than ever.

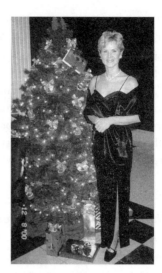

Jeri, who's 59 and lives in Yardley, Pennsylvania, gave up sugar as part of a diet she read about that promised she'd shed 10 pounds in 10 days. The diet required eating steamed vegetables, boiled potatoes, and broiled meats and also giving up sugar, butter, and fried foods. For Jeri, that meant no more of the pies, cakes, and candy that she had always enjoyed.

"I was a big girl, and I didn't like the way my legs rubbed together and the way I couldn't sit down and cross my legs comfortably," says Jeri, who weighed about 160 pounds back then. "Ten days didn't seem like much."

The diet did as it promised, and Jeri lost 10 pounds. Five days into it, she realized she no longer had the sugar cravings she once experienced, the gnawing pangs that would send her running for candy bars and peanut butter crackers. "If I wanted something sweet, I'd just eat fruit," she says.

Ten days soon turned into years, and Jeri gradually lost another 25 pounds. Today, at 5 feet 6 inches tall, she weighs about 125 pounds. She maintains her weight by eating well, teaching aerobics, and remaining sugar-free, refusing even to indulge at a birthday party or wedding.

The rare cravings she gets now are quickly extinguished with a cup of tea, sips of water, or a brisk walk. She is also reminded that both her parents had diabetes and that she used to get migraine headaches from eating sugar. "I ask myself, 'Is that worth it?'" she says. "And that usually keeps me on track."

Telling herself initially that giving up sugar was temporary helped Jeri stop eating sweets for good. "If you say you're going to do this for the rest of your life, it's just too much," she says. "But 10 days isn't so bad. And every day that you don't eat sugar, it becomes easier to just not do it. I think that's good for any kind of nutritional change."

## WINNING ACTION

**Make small changes rather than attempting big ones.** By resolving to go sugar-free for just a couple weeks or cutting out the sweets one at a time, you may be better able to rein in your cravings and ultimately quit sugar for good. In their book, Changing for Good, *authors James O. Prochaska, John C. Norcross, and Carlos C. DiClemente contend that change comes in six stages before a new habit is established, the final stage being termination. Change is maintained, they say, by avoiding tempting situations, creating a new lifestyle, and doing positive thinking.*

# SHE HIRED HELP
# AND DROPPED 35 POUNDS

"I came from a family of 10 kids. My mom totally sugar-loaded the house," confesses Maura O'Connor, a 32-year-old account development manager from Point Lookout, New York. For years Maura, who lived at home until her midtwenties, made a nightly ritual of raiding the family's cupboards for Pop-Tarts, cookies, doughnuts, and sugary cereals.

At 19, the 5-foot-10 Maura weighed 210 pounds and had developed gallstones. When a doctor warned that her weight was putting her health at risk, she undertook the strenuous exercise regimen that she continues to follow today. That includes weight training, running, and Spinning classes 6 or 7 days a week. But she didn't significantly change her eating habits.

"Even as fit as I was, I was still overweight," says Maura. So she tried dieting but found herself bingeing on sweets after dinner. Then in 1997, weighing 200 pounds, she decided to visit a nutritionist. "I had done Weight Watchers for about 10 years, but I felt I wanted a one-on-one approach," she explains.

The nutritionist recommended a 1,300-calorie-a-day diet. She instructed Maura to keep a food diary and to fax a copy to her office twice a week. Over time, Maura began to look at food in a whole new light, thanks to her nutritionist and her food diary. "It makes you accountable for what you're eating," she discovered.

Maura did not immediately change her eating habits. "It took me almost 2 years of seeing a nutritionist to get real with myself and actually take the bad foods out of my diet," she says. "I spent years thinking that working out would justify the desserts and larger portions. I've come to realize you truly are what you eat."

How did she learn that? By paying strict attention to her calorie intake. Now, when she wants dessert after dinner, she checks her food diary. Depending on how many calories she can afford, she allows herself a serving of low-fat ice cream, a Blow Pop, or a handful of pretzels.

Maura's nutritionist—whom she continues to see every other week—provides her with valuable moral support. "It's my own time to talk with her about the way that I feel. She has a true understanding of my diet," explains Maura. "If I get frustrated, she makes me feel better. She tells me, 'Remember how far you've come.'" She also points out weaknesses or strengths in Maura's food diary and recommends methods for sticking to 1,300 calories per day.

Maura worked long and hard at her diet before she finally saw clear results. By May 2000, she'd dropped to 185 pounds. Over the next 6 months, by more strictly maintaining her 1,300-calorie-a-day diet, she shed another 20 pounds, bringing her to her present weight of 165.

### WINNING ACTION

**Work with a nutritionist.** *Got a sweet tooth that just won't quit no matter how hard you try? Consider hiring a nutritionist who can review your diet weekly. A good nutritionist can help you design a healthy diet, coach you through tough times, and make you feel accountable for your food choices. To find a qualified nutritionist, talk to your doctor or call your local hospital for a recommendation. Or check reputable Web sites like the American Dietetic Association's www.eatright.org to tap into their nationwide dietitian referral service.*

# *SMART SHOPPING CUT HER SUGAR INTAKE*

Shellie Winkel initially set out to lose weight, not reduce her sugar consumption. But the more articles and books she read about dieting and proper nutrition, the more wary she became about sugar. "Almost everything I picked up was focusing on sugary foods and other refined carbohydrates, rather than complex carbohydrates like whole grains, fruits, and vegetables," she says.

Shellie started to pay more attention to what she bought at the supermarket. "Anything in a box should be questioned," she says. "People are eating low-fat everything, but they don't realize that often the fat is replaced with sugar." Once she realized this herself, her two to three daily sodas, the cakes, and the cookies all became part of her diet past.

"Now, a normal day for me is oatmeal with fruit for breakfast, a big salad for lunch, and then chicken, steak, or fish for dinner," says Shellie, 37, of Hudson, Wisconsin. "I have protein at lunch and dinner, but I make sure to eat twice as much veggies as protein." She figures that a protein serving is about the size of her palm. For vegetables, she doubles that amount.

White bread also came off Shellie's menu. These days, the only breads she'll eat are items like whole wheat pitas or muffins that she makes herself with whole wheat flour, wheat germ, steel-cut oats, and walnuts, raisins, or bananas. "If I'm going to have bread, it will be healthy and dense with lots of fiber," she says. She also makes her own oatmeal cookies using applesauce or bananas for a sweetener.

Shellie started cutting sugar at the beginning of July 1999, and by the end of August, she had lost 16 pounds. "Once they were gone, I started walking, then running, and now I run all the time," she says. The 5-foot-5 Shellie has since lost another 16 pounds and now weighs 120. "I can wear a size 4, and I'm skinnier than I was before I had my kids."

In addition to shedding those unwanted pounds, Shellie stopped having monthly migraines. "When one came on, all I could do was take medication and lie in bed in a dark, quiet room for up to 2 days," she says. "Once I started cutting out sugar, the migraines went away.

"I feel so much better now—more alert and energetic, stronger, and in control of my life," says Shellie. "At first, it was very hard, almost like I was withdrawing from sugar. Now, I can't handle anything with too much sugar. Even bananas are almost too sweet for me."

Dropping sugar is something Shellie now recommends to everyone. "Some people can do it, and some can't," she says. "But if you just try it, you'll feel better and might even lose weight."

## WINNING ACTION

**Shop the perimeter of the supermarket.** *After all, that's where you'll find basic items—fruit, vegetables, meat, dairy—that provide all the nutrients a body needs. The only sugars are those that occur naturally. The same can't be said of what you'll find lurking in the inner aisles: cake mixes, sugared cereals, jams, jellies, canned fruit in heavy syrup, and acres and acres of soda. Yes, the inner aisles offer some low-sugar foods and baking materials like bran cereal and whole wheat flour, but much of what's there is loaded with sugar. If you watch your step through the market, you've already won a battle against sweets.*

# *SHE LEARNED A LOT BY READING LABELS*

Linda Pase couldn't believe her eyes. But there it was, on the back of her Pepsi.

"There are 41 grams of sugar in just one can!" she says. "I was amazed to learn the amount of sugar in some foods and beverages. And I never realized how much of it I was consuming."

Linda, 47, spends up to 10 hours a day surrounded by sweets, working in the bakery department of a large supermarket. Although she was never tempted by the doughnuts and cookies, she drank a lot of soda—four to five cans a day. "I didn't always have time to get meals, so I would grab a soda when I was hungry," says this resident of Seaford, Delaware.

That was before she invested in a booklet listing the sugar content of foods, which showed her that sugar was hiding in a lot of what she was eating. Based on the booklet's recommendations, she made a point of reading labels and eliminating any food or beverage, including sodas, with more than 3 grams of sugar per serving.

The effort paid off. In September 2000, when Linda made the decision to curtail her sugar consumption, she was carrying 220 pounds on her 5-foot-3 frame. She proceeded to lose nearly 50 pounds in 10 months—18 within the first 2 weeks alone.

"I cannot believe I lost that much weight," she says. "I have always been large, and I've tried every diet and pill known to man. Some plans were too difficult and time-consuming for me to follow; others cost too much. And none of them worked."

What *did* work was paying attention to her sugar intake. Linda says she was surprised by the amount of sugar in foods like dry cereal and even some canned vegetables. "Just get into the habit of reading labels—and if it has more than 3 grams of sugar, don't buy it," she recommends.

Whenever possible, Linda chooses fresh or minimally processed foods, since they tend to have less sugar. She drinks sugar-free soda and uses artificial sweetener in her coffee. And she is spreading the word to her coworkers about checking the sugar content of food. She even convinced several to follow her plan, and all of them have lost weight.

"Others still make fun of me," she says. "But I used to be a size 20, and now I wear size 14. I didn't like being a size 20, and I didn't like the way I looked. Now, I don't mind getting dressed to go out. The shirts I used to wear every day are so big I sleep in them."

## WINNING ACTION

**Read labels for sugar content.** *It's amazing how many people put foods and beverages into their shopping carts without realizing how much sugar these items contain. Sugar isn't just where we expect it, like in soft drinks and candy. It also lurks in foods we consider healthy, such as cereals, yogurt, canned fruit, muffins, and sometimes even canned vegetables. Paying attention to labels is particularly important if you rely on prepared and easy-to-fix foods. Those entrées from the freezer section and that potato salad picked up from the deli may not be as sugar-innocent as you might think. Keep in mind, though, that by avoiding sugary sodas, candy, sweetened baked goods like cookies and cakes, ice cream, and sweetened fruit drinks, you can eliminate much of the added sugar in your diet.*

# *SHE FOUND FREEDOM FROM SUGAR IN FRESH FRUIT*

Greta Heintz has been dieting for most of her 50 years—but she's only recently found the solution to her weight woes. "Whenever I wanted to lose weight, I'd stop eating," she says. "The whole concept of dieting was 'eat less,' so that's what I did, even in the more formal weight-loss programs."

But eating less invariably backfired. "I was hungry because I never ate enough food," says Greta, a professional wedding photographer in Walnut Creek, California. "When I was dieting, I could hold back only so long."

That all changed in June 2000. Three years after her last failed diet, Greta ran across the Pritikin and McDougall programs, both of which came as a shock. They included unlimited whole grains, vegetables, potatoes, and beans and very limited sugar and refined flour. The Pritikin plan also allowed for unlimited whole fruit.

Greta suddenly realized that dieting success might come not from eating less of the same foods you always eat but rather from changing the very foods on your plate. "Prior to this, I had never thought about giving up sugar," she says.

Dropping sugar cold turkey proved rough, but Greta discovered a secret weapon that helped her through. "During the transition period, when I was biting the tabletop to keep from eating sugar, I ate lots and lots of fresh fruit," she says. "Fresh fruit is still my choice if a momentary impulse to eat sugar hits me."

After a week on her new program, the residual urge for sugar seemed to pass from her body, and she was suddenly free—as long as she stuck to a sugar-free diet, that is. If she slipped and nibbled on something sweet, she found herself fighting cravings for at least the next 24 hours.

"The key for me is to avoid sugar altogether," says Greta. "That means no sugar in cereal, no sugar in spaghetti sauce, no sugar in salad dressings. Somehow, fruit doesn't affect me the same way. I can eat fruit, and it doesn't make me want cookies."

Since starting her program, Greta continues to eat six to eight pieces of fruit and six to eight servings of vegetables each day. She prefers fruit in season, such as apples, pears, and bananas in the winter and berries, peaches, and cantaloupe in the summer. She hardly feels like she's dieting at all.

"For the first time, I'm losing weight without deprivation," she says, boasting that she's lost 55 pounds from her 5-foot-7 frame, bringing her down to within 20 pounds of her goal of 145. "Because of the weight loss, I'm way more energetic and capable. I've always walked an hour or more each day, but it's much easier now."

Most important, she doesn't worry anymore that she won't be able to stick with the diet. Says Greta, "I really feel that this is something I can sustain for life."

### WINNING ACTION

**Keep fruit close at hand.** *Yes, raw fruit contains natural sugars, but it also contains numerous health-building vitamins, minerals, and phytochemicals (substances found in plants that can have a beneficial effect on your body)—not to mention fiber, which helps you feel fuller than just a candy bar will. By filling up on fruit, you serve your body much better than starvation does. And with so many fruits available, you're sure to find plenty that suit*

*your taste buds. Head to the produce aisle and start ex-
perimenting.*

## HE GAVE SUGAR THE BOOT
## AND STILL FINDS LIFE SWEET

Like many people approaching middle age, Arnold Mendez found
his weight creeping upward despite his best efforts to stay fit.

"I've exercised since I was a teenager," says Arnold, of Corpus
Christi, Texas. "When I hit 35, I was about 180 to 190 pounds. But
every year after that, I added several pounds, so by the time I was
45, I weighed about 240." Even with daily exercise—he has a black
belt in tae kwon do—and a physically demanding job at the time,
he couldn't seem to slim down. That is, until he read *Sugar Busters!*
and decided to give up sugar.

"I had always known that sugar wasn't the best thing for me,"
says 48-year-old Arnold. But reading the book—and doing additional research while working toward a master's degree in biology
and chemistry—drove the point home. "Sugar is not a naturally occurring substance; it's a refined product made by man. Our bodies
are well-designed, but not well enough to take care of that much
sugar.

"I didn't go on a sugar-free diet—just one free of added sugar,"
adds Arnold. Gone are the couple of Cokes he drank each day as
well as the sweetened iced tea and the sugar added to his cereal or
oatmeal in the morning.

In no way, though, does Arnold feel that he's depriving himself
of sweetness. "I eat a lot of fruit—like dates, grapes, oranges, and
orange juice—and pasta sauce (tomatoes have a lot of sugar in

them)," he says. "I eat a lot of natural sugar, but hardly any white sugar or high-fructose corn syrup."

Arnold says his family has joined him in the diet, and it's easy to see the change in the kitchen. "In a family with three kids, a 5-pound bag of sugar would be gone in a month. Now, I buy a little 1½-pound bag, mostly for guests who want sugar for tea or coffee, and it lasts 4 to 5 months."

Arnold adopted his no-added-sugar diet in early 1999; within 6 months, his weight fell to 197 pounds—healthy for his 5-foot-11 frame. "People think the key to slimming down is exercise, but I think it's diet," he says. "I eat a lot less sugar, and even though I work out less, the weight has come off. Cutting down on sugar has made the difference."

## WINNING ACTION

**Wipe white sugar off your menu.** *Cutting back on your sugar consumption doesn't automatically mean depriving yourself of sweet things. It can be as simple as cutting out a few teaspoons at each meal. Take some off your grapefruit or oatmeal in the morning, out of your coffee at lunch, and out of your iced tea in the evening. If you cut a mere 6 teaspoons per day, you eliminate 100 calories from your meals. What's more, you can double the calorie savings by dropping just one can of regular soda from your daily intake. These small changes add up quickly! Replace the missing sweetness with fruits and naturally sweet vegetables like tomatoes, carrots, and winter squash.*

# *SHE TRICKS HER SUGAR CRAVINGS INTO SUBMISSION*

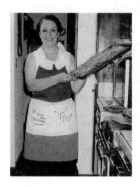

Switching to sugar-free
snacks helped Susan take
off 40 pounds.

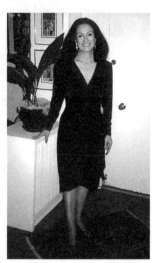

More than 7 years after she
lost 40 pounds, Susan Cursi
still has sugar cravings. But she has learned how to trick them into
believing they are satisfied.

"I eat a sugar-free ice pop," she says. "I especially like the tropical flavors. They are sweet, they are cold, they are very satisfying, and they have only 15 calories."

Susan, 52, hasn't always had such command over her cravings. As an employee in a clothing store, she used to eat what she could, when she could. "It was the 'catch anything you can find to eat' diet," she says: no breakfast, a candy bar for lunch, a second candy bar for midafternoon snack, a heavy dinner, and then bed. At 5 feet 5 inches, she weighed 175 pounds.

"I didn't feel well," says Susan, who lives in Fresno, California.

"I was tired all the time. My father has high blood pressure, and my mother has diabetes—and I saw myself in 5 years having major medical problems. I was eager to change my life."

Susan joined TOPS Club (Take Off Pounds Sensibly), a national weight-loss support group. Within 6 months, she lost 40 pounds.

Along with other dietary changes, she has completely eliminated sugar. True, she allows herself a treat now and then, but only in moderation. "I was at a banquet recently, and they served cheesecake," she says. "I had one bite, and I was satisfied. Before, I would have eaten a whole piece and then looked around for others that I could finish up."

In addition to the frozen pops, Susan keeps sugar-free hard candy and fresh fruit in the house. Strawberries and melon, in particular, satisfy when her sweet tooth acts up.

Susan says that she feels better than she has in years—better even than when she was in high school. She weighed about 160 when she graduated.

"I have more energy than I did then," she says. "My mood is improved. All because of healthy eating."

### WINNING ACTION

**Keep sugar-free treats on hand.** *These foods satisfy the need for something sweet without the sugar that can cause physical reactions, weight gain, and possibly even a full-fledged binge. At the same time, they give your taste buds a happy burst of flavor that's just enough to take the edge off a craving. Sugar-free ice pops are especially refreshing in the summer. Sugarless chewing gum is a good idea for work or when you're otherwise away from home. In addition, gum satisfies the desire to* *chew—a yen that could lead your hands in the direction of the cookie jar if you're not careful.*

# SHE BUYS HER SNACKS BY THE SLICE

Susanne Simmons Sites started gaining weight in her midforties—but that wasn't a problem since she had only 115 pounds on her 5-foot-5½-inch frame. "At first, I was happy," she says. "But within a couple of years, I had gotten up to 161 pounds, and I didn't know how to slim down."

A truck driver at the time, Su-z (as she likes to be known) blamed the weight gain on greasy truck-stop food. "From May 1994 to May 1995, I went low-fat and lost about 30 pounds," says the Las Vegas resident. But by March 1997, she had regained every last ounce.

That summer, she did a lot of swimming, which helped take off the extra pounds. She maintained her weight for 2 years, only to start gaining yet again once she no longer had access to the pool.

Finally, in July 1999, a friend turned Su-z on to the Atkins diet, and she got hooked. "It was really hard the first few months," she says. But before long, she was satisfying her sugar cravings in ways she'd never anticipated. "Instead of ice cream, I ate more chicken, eggs, and hamburger whenever I had a sugar craving," she says.

Chicken and hamburger? Isn't it hard to keep those items handy? Not at all, says Su-z. "It's easy to have the appropriate food available at all times, although it does take planning."

When Su-z started the diet, she worked at an apartment complex cleaning vacated units. "Partway through the morning, I'd open my container of food, usually turkey or chicken, and set it on the counter. Then every time I passed the counter, I'd pop some in my mouth," she says. "Later, when I was driving again, I'd buy precooked meat found in the freezer section, set it on the dash, and munch all day while driving down the road. This kind of eating keeps my blood sugar balanced so I don't have those drastic ups and downs."

After 2 years of low-sugar snacking, 54-year-old Su-z lost those persistent 30 pounds one more time. Now down to 140, she wants to lose 15 to 20 pounds more. "The sugar and carbohydrate addict must think like the recovering alcoholic," says Su-z. "One bite may not hurt, but for the sugar addict, one bite is not enough, just as one drink isn't enough for the alcoholic."

Now that she's gotten sugar out of her life, Su-z can't imagine ever going back. "I feel better, more wide awake, and more energetic than at any other time in my life."

### WINNING ACTION

**Munch on protein instead of sweets.** *Unlike sugary treats that race through your body and send your blood sugar for a loop, a protein-rich snack like lean chicken or turkey or low-fat cottage cheese will keep you on a more even keel—and make you less prone to binge snacking. Since some protein items contain a lot of fat and sodium, be sure to read the labels before you buy to make sure you're not doing your body more harm than good.*

# SHE PUT ON AIRS
# TO STOP EATING SWEETS

With her fortieth high school reunion approaching in October 2001, Beverly Emmons decided to sacrifice her sweet tooth for Lent. "I was eating too much chocolate and not enough good foods," she says. "I figured that if I cut back on chocolate, I might lose some weight, too."

But Beverly didn't want to give up chocolate completely. "I can't totally eliminate sweets from my diet or I will fail," she says. "I decided to make just one change and keep at it until it became a habit."

With that in mind, Beverly decided to turn into a chocolate snob and be very choosy about the types of chocolate that she'll eat. She doesn't feel a need to explain her polite-but-firm refusals. "When others offer me chocolate, I just say, 'No thanks,'" she says.

Those "others" include Beverly's coworkers, who—like coworkers everywhere—maintain a constant flow of sweets in the office. "People bring in lots of things—cookies they baked over the weekend, cake, always something," says Beverly. "We have huge bags of candy, little bite-size things that you take one of, then another, then another."

Once Beverly started upscaling her tastes, though, she found her desire for chocolate becoming more refined. "Thinking about Easter Sunday, I could hardly wait to dig into my grandkids' Easter basket and see what chocolate was there," says the 58-year-old Indianapolis resident. "But when the time came, I was choosier about what I was going to have. There was one dark chocolate in the basket, so I took that and only that."

Months after Lent was over, Beverly realized that the 40-day "training period" had given her the discipline she needed to avoid most sweets. In the process, she lost 15 pounds from her 5-foot-1 frame and weighed in at a comfortable 132. "I'm not eating nearly as much candy as I was before," she says. "Now, it's a choice rather than an uncontrolled urge."

## WINNING ACTION

**Be choosy about chocolate.** Don't settle for what your coworkers bring into the office or what your neighbors offer over the fence. Try to choose a favorite chocolate—one that you can't buy in every market or store—and politely say no to any other kind. As long as you don't rush out and buy a bag of the expensive treats to keep by your side, an elite attitude will help you shun any other chocolate that is dangled in front of your nose.

The same attitude can work for other sweets as well: Latch onto one type of ice cream and refuse any other. Turn aside ordinary sodas in favor of a micro-brewed root beer that's available only at a certain restaurant. Bypass the doughnuts in the supermarket bakery in anticipation of getting your absolute favorite cruller when you go home for the holidays. If you don't settle for inferior sweets, you'll get more enjoyment from the ones you do eat and ensure that you indulge in them only occasionally.

# SHE SWITCHED
# TO SNACK-SIZE TREATS

Bethanny Davis keeps a bag of snack-size candy bars hidden in her house. Every once in a while, when she yearns for chocolate, she pulls out the bag, slips one bar from its wrapper, and eats it. Then she tucks the bag away. She never eats more than one. "It's enough to satisfy my sweet tooth without setting me back too much," says Bethanny, a 29-year-old freelance writer from Casco, Michigan.

Bethanny figures she can spare a small treat now and then. Used to be, she'd snack on a full-size candy bar every morning at 10 A.M. Then she'd lunch on fast food and sip on a 2-liter bottle of Mountain Dew throughout the day.

In January 1999, carrying 180 pounds on her 5-foot-6 frame and none too happy about shopping for size-16 clothes, Bethanny resolved to change. Her goal was to shimmy back into her size 12s again. "I didn't start the diet right away," she says. "First, I spent 2 months deciding how I would do it and talking myself into really doing it." Ultimately, she made up her mind to institute some serious lifestyle changes—changes she could live with. Forever.

Bethanny settled on three major alterations. First, she switched over to diet soda. "It didn't do much to help my caffeine habit, but it sure eliminated a lot of sugar," she observes. In fact, that alone cut a walloping 880 calories from her daily intake. Second, she quit heading out to fast-food restaurants at lunchtime and brought leftovers from home. Third, she began shunning candy bars. She stored grapes in the refrigerator at work and snacked on them when hunger pangs hit.

In 2 months, Bethanny shed 25 pounds, putting her at 155. She's maintained that weight since mid 1999.

Grapes were a terrific alternative to candy bars, Bethanny discovered. But after a while, she found herself craving chocolate again. So she came up with a solution. She bought a bag of snack-size candy bars and decided to eat just one whenever she really wanted chocolate. She hides the bag so it is out of sight and therefore not a constant temptation.

Bethany believes her diet works because she has made changes she is comfortable with. "I love chocolate. Eliminating it completely worked for the first part of my diet, when I initially lost the weight, but I wouldn't want to give it up forever," she asserts.

Today, Bethany wears a size 10, and she's determined to stay there. "It feels good when you look in the mirror and like what you see," she says.

### WINNING ACTION

**Switch to snack-size candy bars.** *Want a smaller-size dress? Choose a smaller-size candy bar. A diet that requires you to forfeit a favorite food, like chocolate, may be destined to fail. Bite-size candy bars, which give you all the flavor of full-size ones for a fraction of the calories, can keep you from feeling deprived and falling off your diet. Store them where they're out of sight and a little inconvenient to get to so you're not tempted to indulge frequently.*

## SHE EATS SWEETS IN SENSIBLE PORTIONS

Fifty-four-year-old Phyllis Ingram has tried many diets over the years, but she's learned that the results from fad diets last only as

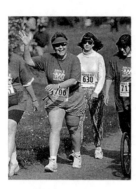

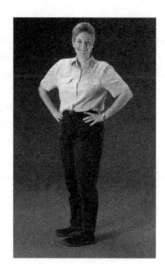

After trying to do without sugar, Phyllis found a way to manage her portions.

long as you actually stick to them—and sometimes not even that long.

"Many people in eating programs feel they have to give something up totally," says Phyllis, who lives in Barto, Pennsylvania. "One time, I went on a sugar-free diet, and I discovered that I couldn't live like that. It's hard in this world of premade, prepackaged supermarket food to get sugar out of your diet. It makes more sense to manage how much sugar you're taking in than to try to purge it completely and live that way."

Since early 2000, Phyllis has been participating in the Weight Watchers Points System, which assigns point values to foods based on their nutritional content. Phyllis is allowed to accumulate a certain number of points over the course of a day, which gives her some freedom in terms of what she eats. "If I do get a sugar craving, I go ahead and eat something," she says. "But I portion it out, so I don't pig out."

To portion her sweets, Phyllis looks for the serving size on a package of sweets and takes exactly that amount—no more. "With Peanut M&M's, for example, I can have about 20 pieces," she says. "Then I try to spread them out over the day so that I don't feel deprived."

Restricting sweets was tough on Phyllis at first, but now it's almost second nature. "In the beginning, it was something I had to concentrate on and talk to myself about. I had to weigh out in my head which treat would be more satisfying: candy throughout the day or a couple of fat-free cookies," says Phyllis. "Now, I go through the day and don't even think about having to choose. As long as I stay within my point range, I can have both."

After a year, Phyllis's new diet system knocked 44 pounds off her 5-foot-6 frame. She's down to 175—and she feels confident that she'll keep losing weight in the future. "This is a dieting method I can do the rest of my life," she says. "I'm not deprived."

### W I N N I N G   A C T I O N

**Spread your sweet supply throughout the day.** *Decide at the start of each day how many sweets you're going to eat, then count or measure out that portion and put the rest out of sight. Perhaps you can eat one sweet every hour or have one at the completion of each project as the day progresses. If you can't wait and you eat everything early, that's too bad—you're still done for the day. Start again tomorrow with your limited supply and try again. Over time, you'll master the art of self-discipline and learn how to keep your sweet tooth in check.*

# *HE WALKED AWAY FROM HIS CRAVINGS*

Robert Fisher can tell you a lot about the cars people drive. That's because he used to pace the parking garage whenever he had a sugar craving.

Robert, who's 54 and lives in Vista, California, gave up eating sugar in 1997. He remembers awaking one Sunday morning after a party, feeling like the proverbial beached whale. Fed up with carrying around extra pounds, he sat down with a pen and paper, drew two circles, and put the foods he ate into two categories: those that satisfied him and those that didn't. The sweet stuff, he realized, never quelled his hunger.

"I also knew that sugar was a major contributor to my not being able to lose weight," Robert says. "I had tried diets, but I realized I had to change my lifestyle."

Robert realized that he had to bid farewell to the doughnuts he ate for breakfast, the candy bars he enjoyed for snacks, and the cake and ice cream he savored at parties. He decided instead to eat more chicken, salads, and tuna. He got in the habit of chucking the top piece of bread on a deli sandwich and ate bran muffins when his officemates were feasting on doughnuts.

"I would always go to sleep somewhat hungry, but when I woke up, I really wasn't very hungry," he says. "I realized my body didn't need to be full all the time."

Early on, the cravings were tough, especially around 3:00 in the afternoon, when Robert was accustomed to grabbing a candy bar. By then, he had already gone through several carrots and pieces of raw cabbage. To calm his cravings, he began taking the elevator to the top floor of the parking garage and winding his way down to the first floor—on foot.

As he walked, he concentrated on his steps and got into a meditative trance. Sometimes, he would look at the thousands of cars parked in the garage. "You start breathing deeply, and you just naturally discourage yourself from eating," he says.

The walks lasted 10 to 15 minutes, enough time to wipe out the craving. Back in his office, Robert would drink a glass of water, then settle back into his work. "Most cravings don't last longer than 10 or 15 minutes anyway," he says. "By then, I'd distracted my body enough to not want the sugar."

Cutting out sweets helped Robert lose 70 pounds in 6 months. At just over 6 feet, he now weighs 170 pounds and sports a 33-inch waist. And he still walks through the parking garage when he has the rare afternoon craving for something sugary.

### WINNING ACTION

**Next time a craving strikes, take a hike.** *Whether you go for a stroll through a parking garage, a nearby park, the office hallways, or your neighborhood, you'll distract yourself for just enough time to let the craving pass. Walking also perks up your energy level, burns some calories, and tones your legs, so you'll be doing a lot more than just dodging a craving.*

## HE KEPT HIS GOAL IN SIGHT—LITERALLY

Joe Dougherty was fed up. At 6 feet 2 inches, he weighed 202 pounds, nearly 20 pounds more than he should have.

And he was nearing 39, the age at which his father had died suddenly of a heart attack. "He was taking down Christmas lights," recalls Joe, who was 10 when his father passed away. "The doctor says that he was dead before he hit the floor.

"I didn't want to end up like that," he adds. "I decided that I was making a permanent change."

But he needed an incentive—something to convince him to forgo the breakfast bar and hot chocolate in the morning and the vending-machine snack at midafternoon. So he turned to his old clothes.

"I have an old pair of shorts that I really like but that I couldn't button anymore," says Joe, who lives in Herndon, Virginia. "I put them out by the bed, so I would see them in the morning and at night. This was on January 2, 2001, exactly 25 years to the day my father died. They got me into the right mind-set."

Four months later, Joe had slimmed down to 181 pounds. He could run with the members of the soccer team he coaches and take the steps at work two at a time.

And he could wear those shorts.

Joe, who does media relations for a think tank in Washington, D.C., says that long afternoons at the office were his worst times for sugar cravings. "I felt like I had to have what I called brain food," he says. "Something cold and sweet and something chocolate. It was a daily habit."

At night, after his three children were in bed, he would relax with a book, television, or conversation. And cups of heavily sweetened tea. "I wouldn't even count the sugar by teaspoons but by seconds that I held the container upside down," he says.

Now, the afternoon snacks have been replaced by drinks of cold water or, for a treat, diet soda. His nighttime tea, if he has it at all, is sweetened with a sugar substitute. Joe has also traded sugar-laden temptations such as cake and ice cream for healthy, naturally sweet snacks such as fruit. He might indulge on special occasions, but even then, he consumes a lot less than he used to. As a result, he relishes those treats even more.

Joe, who's now 36, says he will be able to stick with his new diet. The afternoon snacks no longer call to him.

"I have lost the cravings," he says. "At this very minute a year ago, I would have been down at the snack machine. Now, I have no desire for anything in there."

### W I N N I N G   A C T I O N

***Put out favorite, too-small clothes as a reminder of where you want to be.*** *Nothing is a better indication that we have gained a few pounds than a snug waistband. Nothing is more gratifying than finally fitting into a favorite garment that was too small. By keeping it out where you can see it, you're sure to start and end each day with a solid reminder of the reason that sugar is no longer a part of your diet.*

## WITH GOOD PLANNING, SHE WIPED SUGAR OFF THE MENU

Some people don't know what they're having for dinner until an hour before they sit down at the table. Sabrina Baker knows a week in advance. By planning her meals ahead of time, Sabrina gave her diet the structure she needed to overcome a lifelong sweet tooth.

Sabrina's passion for sugar started early. As an infant, she rejected her mother's breast milk in favor of orange juice. As an adult, she ate chocolate almost every day, had desserts at lunch and dinner, and once considered starting a business making truffles. "I nibbled on chocolate after dinner, and I looked for reasons to make cakes, cookies, truffles, and candies," says Sabrina, a 29-year-old Seattle resident. "If there were cookies around the house, I ate them all day long."

In March 2000, Sabrina decided to quit her sugar habit. At the time, she was plagued by achy joints, frequent headaches, and constant fatigue. Her naturopathic doctor advised her to give up wheat as well as white flour and sugar.

"I had tried to quit sugar a few months before that, but within a week or two, I'd break down," she says. "But having a doctor tell me to do it was a challenge, and I was ready for it."

Sabrina stopped making sweets for herself and started reading labels to avoid buying sugar-laden foods. She replaced her morning muffins with oatmeal and blueberries, switched from peanut butter to cashew butter, and ate fruit in place of sugary snacks. To satisfy cravings, she chose bananas or protein foods, such as nuts, over something sweet.

"The first 2 weeks were total hell," Sabrina admits. "I was having dreams of cakes falling through the air. It felt like withdrawal from a drug."

With encouragement from her husband and the help of a software program called AccuChef, Sabrina adopted a whole new approach to eating. Using AccuChef, she'd select and print out recipes for an entire week's worth of dinners. The program provided a shopping list of recipe ingredients, which Sabrina took to the grocery store. She'd plan most lunches and snacks, too.

"This has saved us a lot of time and money," Sabrina says. "But it's also enabled me to be more disciplined about my diet."

That kind of discipline gave Sabrina the structure she needed to give up sugar, which she credits with eliminating her headaches, joint pain, and fatigue. It also helped her shed 15 pounds from her 5-foot-4 frame. She now weighs 125. "Nobody believes me when I tell them that sugar makes them fat," she says. "But I can tell you that it does."

## WINNING ACTION

**Plan your meals ahead of time.** *Knowing what you'll eat at each meal puts you in control and leaves you less likely to get sidetracked into a sugar fest when hunger overrides your good judgment and good intentions. Write down your menus, then grocery shop according to those plans. You'll be less apt to pick up unplanned sweets and more likely to buy the wholesome, healthy foods that will do your body good. As a bonus, you'll save time and money by cutting back on last-minute trips to the store and expensive impulse items.*

# A LATE LUNCH THROWS HER CRAVINGS OFF SCHEDULE

Every day around 3 P.M., Danielle Pagano used to join her colleagues for a coffee break that typically included cookies or brownies. But when she started eating a late lunch and limiting desserts to special outings, Danielle wiped out her mid-afternoon sugar cravings and eventually lost 30 pounds.

Danielle, who's 31 and lives in Hoboken, New Jersey, first began evaluating her sugar intake when she got engaged in 1999. At 5 feet 6 inches tall, she weighed 155 pounds and wanted to slim down for the wedding. "Like every good bride, I wanted to lose weight," she says. "But instead of going on one of these crash diets, I decided to learn to eat better once and for all."

A visit to a nutritionist helped her realize she was a carbohydrate junkie who loved pizza, bagels, and breads. She followed most meals with dessert and took time every workday afternoon to feast on cookies and brownies. Sometimes, she had a snack between breakfast and lunch, too, albeit a healthier one such as granola.

Danielle began to change not only what she ate but also when she ate. She cut out all starches and sugars and focused on vegetables, fruits, and grains. Instead of eating a bagel for breakfast, she had whole-grain cereal, a banana, and fat-free milk. But she didn't eat it until she got to work at 9 A.M. The late breakfast made it easier for her to postpone lunch until 2 P.M., when she usually had a salad with grilled chicken or a sandwich with half the bread.

"By eating lunch at 2, I had no opportunity for hunger in the late afternoon," she says. "Now, sometimes, it doesn't even occur to me to eat, and I'll say, 'Wow, it's 2:00.'" She says it also helps that she has a very busy job as a marketing manager for mutual funds.

The effort turned Danielle into a more svelte bride. By the time she got married 10 months after she started the diet, she had shed 30 pounds and weighed 125. And she has kept herself around 130 since then, thanks to the healthier diet and regular workouts at the gym.

Now when the 3:00 break comes along, Danielle no longer heads out with her colleagues. She still enjoys an occasional dessert when she goes out to dinner but usually shares it with her companion or just takes a few bites. And when she has a craving for pizza, Danielle allows herself a slice—with no remorse. "Once you get things under control, you can allow yourself the occasional treat," she says.

*W I N N I N G   A C T I O N*

**Eat a later lunch to avoid afternoon snacking.** *By postponing lunch until a little later in the day—and making sure it's a healthy meal—you'll head off the afternoon munchies. That's especially important if your usual inclination is to reach for something sugary around 3:00. By the time you're hungry again after your late lunch, you'll be home from work and ready for a sensible dinner.*

## SHE KEEPS FRESH VEGGIES AT HER FINGERTIPS

Roe WiersGalla used to stash her favorite gourmet chocolates in her desk drawer. But these days, the chocolate has been replaced by a container of fresh vegetables. Now when she gets a craving for something sweet, Roe munches on carrots, broccoli, cauliflower, celery, or brussels sprouts that have been cooked and chilled.

Roe, who's 56 and lives in Milwaukee, was a lifelong devotee of sweets. Cakes were her favorite, but she also loved candy, cookies, ice cream, and pudding. After years of eating with reckless abandon, Roe—who's 5 feet 2 inches—hit her peak weight of 365 pounds. Still, she did nothing to change her eating habits. She simply bought cars that could accommodate her size, parked in the closest parking spots, and had her clothing custom-made. "It was just more fun to

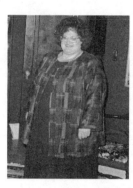

A secret stash of veggies helped Roe lose 175 pounds—and keep them off.

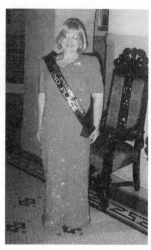

eat," she says. "I had pretty much resolved that I was going to die weighing 400 pounds."

That changed when Roe discovered she had peripheral vascular disease, a condition that causes narrowing and hardening of the arteries in the legs and feet and prevents oxygen and blood from reaching body tissues. In January 1997, Roe joined Take Off Pounds Sensibly (TOPS Club), began seeing a nutritionist, and took up walking. While she dieted, she ate an occasional sweet but always stayed within her calorie limits.

By November 1998, Roe had slimmed down to 190 pounds—10 pounds below her goal. That's when she lost control. "Hearing the doctor tell me I didn't have to lose any more weight was like getting a green light," she says. "I started to eat indiscriminately."

One day, she managed to devour 5,000 calories' worth of cake, cookies, candy, and ice cream, beginning with four pieces of carrot cake in the morning. That's when Roe put on the brakes. The next day, March 23, 1999, she decided to have no sweets at all. She tried the same thing the next day and the next. She has not eaten a single dessert since.

To stifle her cravings, Roe bought cut vegetables and put them in a 1-pound margarine container in her desk drawer. Whenever she felt the urge to eat, she crunched on veggies instead. "I usually start nibbling around 10:30 in the morning," she says. "I'll have a healthy lunch, and then I nibble throughout the afternoon. The veggies satisfy my grazing needs." She also takes the veggies on road trips and carries fruit—apples, bananas, pears, cherries, and grapes—with her in her bag.

Keeping old photos of herself on her desk, on the refrigerator, and in front of her treadmill in the basement helps her stay inspired, too. "Those photos remind me of how limited my life was back then," she says.

Roe, who is holding steady at 190 pounds, admits she misses eating desserts but doesn't think she'll ever go back to them. "Now, I can actually look at a gorgeous display case of desserts and admire them," she says. "It's sort of like looking at my boss's Ferrari. They're beautiful, but I'm not going to have one."

### WINNING ACTION

**Keep cut-up vegetables within easy reach for a quick snack.** You may find that your urge to eat something sweet is actually an urge for an oral fix, which you can easily satisfy with crunchy veggies. And there's so much more to choose from than old standby celery. Baby carrots are especially fun, but broccoli and cauliflower florets, radishes, sugar snap peas, bell peppers, and jicama are equally satisfying. Check the supermarket for other ideas. If you select ready-cut vegetables in the produce *section or from the salad bar, it will be that much more convenient to sustain the habit.*

## HE JUICED UP HIS DIET TO SHED THE EXTRA POUNDS

Bill Whedon permits himself the occasional chocolate—"one or two pieces a month," he says. But before indulging, he reaches for a 10-ounce glass of carrot juice or orange juice. Often, the juice chases off the yearning for chocolate.

"It kind of satisfies the craving for sweet stuff," says Bill, who's 58 and lives in Lawson, Missouri. "You get good sugar flavor, and it enters the bloodstream at a low rate," which prevents an immediate sugar high and subsequent plunge, he says.

But Bill hasn't always been so careful about what he ate. In 1991, his weight hit a high of 260 pounds. At 5 feet 10 inches, his body was 32 percent fat. But he wasn't worried. "I always felt that I was in good shape," he says. "I was just a big boy."

Then a friend convinced him to go to the gym for an aerobics class. "I got so winded in just 10 minutes I couldn't go any further," Bill says. "I started paying attention to my health then."

That meant pancakes "loaded up with syrup" were off the menu. Sodas, pastries, and desserts were also gone, replaced with fresh fruits, juices, and yogurt. Red meat gave way to tofu, chicken, and salmon.

Bill also started exercising 4 or 5 days a week, usually choosing between walking and high-impact aerobics. "I just quit being a slothful pig," he says. After 1 year, his weight dropped to 165 pounds, and his body fat to 16 percent. In the 10 years since, his weight has averaged 180 and his body fat 18 percent.

In addition to getting him into shape, exercise helped Bill avoid the sweets he so loved. "Sweets tended to weigh me down," he says. "I had to feel good when I was exercising, so I got out of the habit of eating sugary stuff."

Bill believes that he got his eating under control just in time. Four years after he started his diet, a family member who weighed 400 pounds rolled over onto his back while sleeping and choked to death. In 2000, Bill himself developed uncontrolled angina and underwent surgery. The doctor told him that if he hadn't been in such good shape, he probably would not have survived the experience.

"I am three times more fit than I was at age 48, two times more fit than at 28 or 38," Bill says. "I feel incredible. I feel a lot better about myself."

## WINNING ACTION

***If you want juice, be choosy.*** *True, fruit juices are much more nutritious than most sweets. So if you've got to satisfy your sweet tooth, a glass of juice might be your best bet. Just be sure to read labels and choose a brand that delivers a relatively small number of calories and grams of sugar per serving. Try diluting half a serving with sparkling water, experimenting with proportions to get the right mix of flavor and fizz. Better yet, make your own juice. Fresh-squeezed can have a lot of sugar, too— but it's natural, compared with the added sugars common in commercial brands.*

# *HE DRINKS HIS TEA SUGAR-FREE*

Don't ask Graham Foat if he wants one lump or two. He takes his tea sugar-free, thank you very much.

Used to be, the 48-year-old marketing and communications consultant from Ilford, England, automatically added a spoonful of sugar to all his hot drinks. That meant he'd swallow 2 or 3 heaping teaspoons of white stuff a day.

Back in 1995, at the urging of some friends and in the interest of maintaining his health, Graham decided to tame his sweet tooth—at least as far as hot drinks were concerned. His first attempt lasted about 3 months. "During those months, I put up with the taste of sugar-free tea and coffee. I never really got used to it, and I eventually went back to using sugar," he says.

Then, several months later, a friend served him a cup of tea that Graham assumed was sugarless. "I thought I might just as well drink it, and I struggled through heroically. Imagine my delight when I reached some super-sweet dregs and realized that they *had* put in the sugar but just hadn't stirred it! My endurance was rewarded, and an idea was born."

His epiphany? To add just half a teaspoon of sugar but plunk down his spoon without stirring—then drink his tea unsweetened until he savored the final syrupy sips. By so doing, he could experience a burst of sweetness with only half the sugar. "You'd be surprised how effective that reward is at getting you through the ordeal," he says.

Soon, Graham began working to cut back even more. He found that just one sip of sugary tea or coffee was enough to balance out the sugar-free part. So he opted to stop drinking the moment he detected the first trace of sugar. After about 4 months, he'd become so accustomed to unsweetened tea that he eliminated sugar completely from his drinks. He's made a habit of passing on it ever since.

Nevertheless, Graham hadn't completely won the sugar war. He liked candy and snacked on a chocolate bar every day. Then, in February 2001, carrying 227 pounds on his 6-foot frame, he decided to trim down. Using the Weight Watchers Points System, Graham became aware of how many calories those candy bars were costing him.

"I don't eat them anymore because I can see a very specific link between chocolate bars and weight gain that I hadn't appreciated before," he says. By counting calories and swearing off sweets, Graham dropped 25 pounds in 4 months, taking him to 203 pounds and closer to his target weight of 170. He's glad he quit stirring his tea all those years ago. "If I hadn't, I guess I would have put on even more weight," he says.

### WINNING ACTION

**Take your coffee or tea sans sugar.** *Graham spent months weaning himself from the flavor of sweetened hot drinks. Here's why you should too: One level teaspoon of the white granules equals approximately 5 grams; a rounded teaspoon, even more. Not much if you have only a cup a day. But multiply that by three and you've sipped down at least 15 grams of sugar and 60 unnecessary calories. Imagine how the calories add up if you do that every day for years on end.*

## SHE THREW OUT THE SUGAR BUT KEPT THE SWEETNESS

Carol Doersom used to work as a decorator for a man who brought doughnuts in nearly every morning to share with both customers and staff. "Eight years and about 1,500 doughnuts later, I was 25 pounds heavier and gaining about a pound a month," says Carol, who lives in Houston.

But when she outgrew a pair of new, larger pants that she had purchased just a few weeks earlier, Carol knew it was time to get her sweet tooth under control.

Since that day in late 1999, Carol has cut sugar and most other carbohydrates out of her diet almost completely. She cooks more often and eats out less to have more control over her meals. And she shops the perimeter of the supermarket for fresh foods instead of buying the processed items that haunt the interior aisles.

But Carol's sugar-busting ways haven't kept her away from desserts, since she's managed to incorporate sugar substitutes into her cooking. "I must have dessert once a day or I feel deprived," she says. "It's always homemade, using the sugar substitute sucralose instead of sugar. I never buy packaged desserts anymore, and knowing that I can whip up something yummy at home is usually enough to keep me from ordering dessert at a restaurant.

"Chocolate mousse is my standby," says Carol, who's now 50. "I make it by mixing ricotta, sour cream, whipping cream, cocoa, vanilla, and sucralose. It's quick and easy, and it tastes great. My husband is addicted to the stuff."

Carol also makes ice cream occasionally by using cream, egg substitute, amaretto, and protein powder. "There are lots of recipes for ice cream on the Internet," she says. "Lately, I've used plain yogurt with sucralose and the juice of a couple of lemons to make something a lot like an Italian ice. Fresh berries on top are nice when they're in season."

Since cutting the sugar from her diet, Carol—who's 5 foot 2—has dropped from 131 pounds to 112. "In addition to losing weight," she says, "a 2-year yeast infection disappeared within a week, and I don't have to nap anymore during the day or in the evening."

The bottom line, says Carol, is that "I've eaten less sugar in a year and a half than I was eating before in a typical day."

*WINNING ACTION*

**Use sugar substitutes when you cook.** *You're not interested in the calories that sugar provides—only the sweetness. There are a number of products on the market—such as aspartame, acesulfame-K, saccharin, and sucralose—that can be used in place of sugar. These sweeteners are often sweeter than sugar itself, so it may take you some time to adjust your recipes. With practice, though, you'll be turning out sugar-free treats that taste identical to your desserts of old! Be sure to read the labels to find out which substitutes can withstand the heat of cooking and baking and which are best for uncooked foods only.*

## *DESSERT LEAVES WHEN HER VISITORS DO*

When Ruby Goldsmith hosts a party, her guests leave with something sweet. That's because 60-year-old Ruby gets rid of leftover desserts by giving them away. It's one way Ruby keeps her house a sugar-free zone. "I know a lot of people who have a sweet tooth," she says. "They'd rather skip dinner and eat dessert."

Not long ago, Ruby was just as passionate about sweets, especially cakes, candy, cookies, and ice cream. "Once I had them in the house, I wouldn't stop eating them until they were finished," says Ruby, who lives near Toronto.

Her love of anything sweet was rooted in her Northern Ireland upbringing, where a cup of tea was always accompanied by a cookie. As an adult, she drank a lot of Coca-Cola and loved sugary breakfast cereals. "Instead of eating potato chips, I'd have a bowl of cereal and tell myself that was okay," says Ruby. "I didn't realize how much sugar I was getting."

In 1988, Ruby was diagnosed with diabetes, a disease that ran in her mother's family. Ruby decided to stop eating sugar in the hopes of reining in her blood sugar levels. She read articles about sugar and became better educated about nutrition labels. She stopped bringing sugary foods into her home and substituted sugar-free hard candies for the sugared ones. She also ate more fruits, vegetables, and whole grains and took up roller-skating and baseball. "It was really hard at first," she says. "But as long as I kept busy, I could be distracted from sugar and sweets."

But since she enjoys entertaining twice a month, Ruby didn't want to deprive her guests of dessert. So she learned to pass along any unfinished sweets, such as double-fudge cake, that made their way into her house. "If a cake or pie is not eaten, then my guests get it," she says. "It's the best way I can find to entertain people and not eat all the leftovers."

Ruby still enjoys an occasional slice of cake or pie, but for the most part, she has eliminated sugar from her diet. Going sugar-free has also helped Ruby shed 80 pounds from her 5-foot-2 frame; she now weighs 130. Her diabetes is also under control. "Giving up sugar has helped me in many ways," she says. "I don't feel as tired, and I still have my own teeth!"

# SHE ATE PIES AND PUDDINGS AND LOST 40 POUNDS

Katrina Martin loves desserts. Pies, puddings, and luscious sweet drinks are all hard and fast favorites of hers. She has them often and even claims they helped her shed 40 pounds from her 5-foot-4 frame.

How is that possible? Katrina prepares all her desserts from scratch, using recipes that she sweetens only with fruit, never with refined sugar. "I've learned some of the wondrous possibilities of fruit," says the 26-year-old customer service coordinator from Oakland, California.

There was a time when packaged cupcakes served as her main source of sustenance. "Oh, God, was I a binger!" confesses the now-reformed Katrina. "I would eat Hostess Sno Balls like they were going out of style. And any kind of chocolate. And white bread. I would eat loads of these foods every single day."

She put an end to that in December 2000, when she vowed to relinquish refined sugar and flour. Despite being a vegan who eschewed meat, milk, and eggs, she was, at that time, about 50 pounds overweight. She'd quit smoking the month before, and her sugar cravings, always strong, had gone haywire. "I tried to control them, but it was futile," she comments.

So Katrina opted for more drastic measures. After going on a 10-day juice fast (which should be done only under a doctor's care), she set about "retraining" her body to tolerate solid foods again. She scoured the Internet for tasty recipes that used no refined sugar or white flour, both triggers that caused her to eat more and more. She ended up filling a three-ring binder with the mouthwatering entrée and dessert recipes she collected.

"I have found a way to make foods that taste sinfully delicious to me," reveals Katrina. Salsa and garlic have replaced sugar and salt as her choice seasonings for main dishes. Fruit-based desserts pacify her sweet tooth. Using her juicer ("It's the best $189 investment I ever made"), Katrina concocts a variety of scrumptious drinks. A favorite calls for blending together one pineapple and one pint of strawberries. "It's like a Creamsicle in a glass," she swears.

She also makes a healthful pancake batter by tossing half a banana, 1 cup of rolled oats, 1 cup of water, and 1 teaspoon of baking powder into a blender. And a pudding with dates, fresh coconut, and vanilla extract. Katrina even whips up a pumpkin pie using sugar-free graham crackers for a crust and substituting pitted dates, the sweetener stevia, and tofu for sugar and milk. "Guaranteed to be the hit of any party!" she says.

Katrina, who still aims to lose 10 pounds to bring her down to 144, doesn't think about cupcakes and candy bars anymore. "It was terribly difficult at first," she admits. "But eventually, I missed sugar less and less until the cravings, for the most part, disappeared."

# SHE NIXED JUICE AND JELLY BEANS TO GET BACK TO A SIZE 6

In 1998, when Mary Launi was pregnant with her daughter, her doctor informed her that she was gaining too much weight. Mary was surprised. She proudly announced she'd been eating healthy foods, including drinking a 16-ounce bottle of orange juice or cranberry juice every morning. "Right away, my doctor told me to cut out the juice, that it was loaded with sugar and was most likely the source of my weight gain," says Mary, 35, a former ad agency art buyer and now a full-time homemaker from Westmont, Illinois.

"I was so shocked," Mary recalls. "I grew up drinking juice, thinking it was healthy." That's when Mary began avidly watching her sugar intake. She'd already been careful about added fats and tried to stick to low-fat desserts. But when she looked at the nutrition label on the fat-free brownies she loved, she found that each

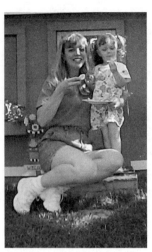

Mary is raising her daughter to be smart about sweets.

one had a walloping 24 grams of sugar—almost equal to 6 teaspoons. "After that, I started checking the sugar in all foods that were low-fat or no-fat," she says.

What she found was that many foods, like yogurt, are loaded with sugar. And fat-free candies like jelly beans and licorice? She ate them by the bagful until she realized, during her pregnancy, that all that sugar was just being converted into fat anyhow.

Now, she reminds herself of that often. "Every time I go to the grocery store, I tell myself that these high-sugar items are fat," she says. "If you have it, I tell myself, your body will just turn it into fat." Keeping that in the forefront of her mind helps her, more often than not, win what she calls "a constant battle of wills."

It enables her to pass by the red licorice twists at the supermarket and pull snacks like popcorn and pretzels and fruits like watermelon from the shelves instead. It encourages her to ignore the juice aisle completely. In fact, she's been careful to avoid giving her 3-year-old daughter any juice at all to keep her from developing a taste for sugar. Both mother and daughter drink water and milk almost exclusively. "To get the vitamins, we'll just eat an orange or an apple instead of drinking juice," she says.

Mary, who is 5 feet 8 inches tall, gained 50 pounds during her pregnancy. She lost 20 after the birth but still had 30 to shed. It took her about a year of exercise (she jogs daily) and dieting to get back to her size-6 clothes. She's been wearing them since 1999.

*WINNING ACTION*

**Remind yourself that excess sugar turns into fat.** *This is not an easy concept to grasp. We've become so attuned to cutting fat from our diets that we forget extra calories from anything—including fat-free sugary foods—are stored by the body as fat. So next time you shop, don't be so considerate of your sweet tooth. Think of your thighs! Your waist! Your health! Check nutrition labels to ferret out foods that are too high in sugar and leave them at the store. Knowing that sugar eventually becomes body fat makes sweets much less appealing and easier to pass up.*

# HE WORKED THE SUGAR OUT OF HIS SYSTEM

When Cesar Mogollon was growing up, his family indulged in sweets after every meal—and sometimes in place of the meal. "In the morning, sweets were okay by themselves," he says. "You didn't need to have a traditional breakfast as long as you had some sweet bread or a doughnut . . . or several doughnuts."

As a result, Cesar was somewhat heavy throughout his teens and into adulthood. "I always topped a meal off with dessert, whether it was some type of pastry, pie, cake, or ice cream," he says. "It was anything and everything."

Cesar was diagnosed with hyperthyroidism in his twenties, so despite his passion for sweets (and fatty fried foods), his metabolism ran so high that he stayed in relatively good shape.

Until May 1993, that is, when he suffered a thyroid storm that sent him to intensive care for a week with a 105-degree temperature. The hospital treated him to reduce the size of his thyroid, which solved one problem. Unfortunately, with his metabolism running at normal speed, Cesar had a new problem to deal with: "After 5 months of denial, eating whatever and whenever I wanted, I ballooned up to 297 pounds."

Finally, Cesar accepted that he could no longer eat like he once did. He had to eliminate the sweets, the soda, the beer, the junk food—"either that or not live too long, basically." But he didn't think a diet alone would be enough, so at the beginning of November, he started attending a local gym.

"I was so motivated by the workouts that my natural inclination was not to touch anything bad for me," says Cesar. "It took 3 weeks to see any kind of result, but then the weight came off like water, and I intensified the exercise."

The workouts were so time-intensive that he had few moments to contemplate eating sweets. He would ride the stationary bike for an hour, then go on to the weight machines. "I supplemented that with as many sit-ups as I could do in a given amount of time, usually between 100 and 500 every morning," he says. By April 1994, he had dropped to 172 pounds on his 6-foot-1 frame.

Over the past few years, Cesar, now 36, has reduced his exercise to 2 days per week and maintained his weight at 190 pounds. Although he snacks occasionally with his sons, he's kept to a low-sugar, low-fat diet. "Ice cream or yogurt probably once a week is about it," says the Palmdale, California, resident. "When we go to buffets, I try to fill myself up with other foods before I even get to that point. I end up feeling better for it."

### WINNING ACTION

**Exercise to distract yourself.** *Don't give in to your cravings right away. When the longing for a sweet hits you, perform some set amount of exercise—perhaps 15 minutes of hand weights and aerobics, two laps around your block, 40 sit-ups, whatever seems appropriate—before you consider yielding to the desire. If you still want the sweet after the workout, at least you're rewarding yourself for work done—and calories burned—rather than downing calories that might become your lifelong companions.*

## SHE HIT THE GYM AND GOT THIN

Back in 1996, Cecilia Fallert was charged with organizing a fitness program for her coworkers. The 54-year-old community newspaper editor introduced a 9-week system, developed by a local hospital, which gave points for exercising and eating healthy foods. By the end of the challenge, Cecilia, who's 5 feet 7 inches tall, had shed 15 pounds, dropping from 175 to 160. Trouble is, within a year, she gained back every ounce. And she knew why: Once the program ended, she couldn't continue her efforts on her own.

In 1998, she was still carrying around that extra weight when a new gym opened in the town of Perryville, Missouri, where she lives. A friend suggested she and Cecilia join together. Cecilia had never before committed herself to a formal exercise routine. "But I wasn't really happy with myself," she recalls. So she joined. Once she'd begun working out regularly, however, she noticed that many women at the gym were still overweight. "I felt that if I wanted to get the most out of my exercise, I had to change the way I was eating," says Cecilia.

A busy woman constantly under deadline, Cecilia relied almost daily on large candy bars and packaged brownies for bursts of energy. She frequently downed doughnuts for breakfast and ended dinner with dessert. Her three weekly sessions at the gym inspired her to change all that. "I don't think you can exercise without dieting or at least without eating good food," she decided. She dusted off the program she'd followed during the office challenge 2 years before and began eating a balanced diet full of fruits and vegetables and keeping sweets and fatty foods to a minimum.

Forgoing her daily dose of sugar was tough at first. "It's kind of like quitting smoking," notes Cecilia, who had given up cigarettes prior to dieting. She broke off slowly, allowing herself, during the first month, one Godiva chocolate at the end of each day. She also began stocking her office refrigerator with baby carrots, whole wheat bread, and blueberries or other fruits—a habit she continues to follow today. Three days a week, when the paper comes out, she's too busy for lunch. "I eat whole wheat cereal in the morning and graze on fruits and vegetables all through the day," she says.

She always finds time to exercise, visiting the gym three times a week for a 40-minute session that includes 10 minutes of stretching and 30 minutes of hydraulic resistance. "It helps to go to the gym because you can see other people around you trying to stay fit," she observes.

The effort proved worthwhile. Cecilia lost 35 pounds in 6 months. She regained 15 and finally found her comfortable weight of 145, which she has maintained since 1999.

*WINNING ACTION*

***Join a gym.*** *Can't seem to find the motivation to sustain a low-sugar diet? Joining a gym could help. It will encourage you to establish a regular exercise routine. Then, you can convince yourself not to sabotage your efforts by snacking on sugary foods. What's more, spending time at a gym allows you to surround yourself with other fitness-minded people, which is bound to keep you inspired.*

## SHE STAYS FOCUSED WITH PHOTOS

Anne Washburn keeps a photo of herself in her purse. It was taken on July 4, 2000, back when she weighed 230 pounds. "Whenever I'm rummaging in my purse, I see it and I think, 'Oh, I can't believe I ever looked like that!'" says Anne, a 25-year-old public relations account executive who resides in Coral Gables, Florida. That photo and others have helped inspire Anne to maintain a diet that allows almost no sugars.

Anne, who's 5 feet 10 inches tall, began putting on weight after puberty. Throughout her early twenties, she regularly gave in to sugar cravings. "I would be lying in bed at night and start thinking about ice cream," she says. "I would get up, get dressed, get into my car, and drive down to the store to buy ice cream."

She admits she wasn't careful about what she ate at other times either. She downed sugary soft drinks daily and snacked on cakes and cookies at the office. Ice cream was her biggest weakness. "I would think, 'What's one more scoop of ice cream? I'm already fat,'" she explains.

But in September 2000, after a doctor told her she ought to lose weight to avoid otherwise inevitable knee and back problems, Anne decided to check out the Atkins diet. She was skeptical about the author's assertion that if you stop eating sugar, you'll stop craving it, but she thought it was worth a try. She eliminated almost all carbs, including sugars, from her diet, nixing even fruit. She began snacking on things like olives and peanuts and dining on soups, salads, steamed vegetables, and meats. Early on, she found herself longing for ice cream. Deeply determined, she willed herself to resist temptation. "You just have to continually say no to yourself," she insists.

Anne says she was surprised when the diet actually worked and she began dropping about 2 pounds a week. Then, in December, 3 months after her diet had begun, a coworker brought in pictures from a Fourth of July gathering. By that time, Anne was 20 pounds lighter than she'd been in the photos, and she was surprised at how heavy she'd looked. She kept one of the pictures and slipped it into her purse. Then she set up a few other pictures of her "fat" self. "I keep one in my house, one in my car, one in my office, one in my purse," she says. "I don't actively look at them, but I have them around." They serve as concrete proof that her diet is well worth the effort and add to her determination to resist sweets.

Within 7 months, Anne shed 45 pounds and slimmed down from a size 22 to a size 14. Today, she weighs 185 pounds and is working on losing another 20 pounds. Does she still suffer from sugar cravings? Not as badly, and when she does, she never gives in to them. "I really like the way I look now," she says.

# SHE CONVINCED HERSELF OF SUGAR'S EVILS

Loretta Killian was a self-described junk food junkie who could down a six-pack of Pepsi in a day, a dozen cookies in a sitting, or three-quarters of a chocolate cake in an afternoon. But it wasn't until she told herself sugar was "poisonous" that she was able to walk away from sweets.

As a teenager, Loretta found that junk food had no effect on her weight. An addiction to recreational drugs prevented her from putting on pounds. But when Loretta stopped using drugs in the late 1970s, her cravings for sugar intensified, and the weight piled on. "I gained 30 pounds almost overnight, and all my clothes were splitting at the seams," says the 44-year-old resident of Reading, Pennsylvania.

Loretta had traded one addiction for another, one that she says was even more potent. "With drugs, it was just a matter of staying

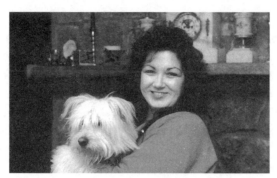

A bit of negative thinking kept Loretta away from sweets.

away from certain people," she says. "But it was hard to get away from sugar. Sugar was like alcohol to me."

Six months after quitting the drugs cold turkey, Loretta went after her sugar habit. She was tired of feeling groggy and lethargic, spending her days in a bathrobe, and at 170 pounds, weighing more than she should. She began eating a high-protein diet and diligently planning every meal. At the start of each day, she wrote in a notebook what she was going to eat, along with her day's activities, reading, and chores. And at the top of the page, she always wrote, "Sugar is poison."

"Whenever I had a sugar craving, I'd just look in my book," she says. "It was like an affirmation, and it worked for me."

In just 3 days, Loretta started feeling better. She could think more clearly, and she felt more energetic than she had in years. The cravings for sugar quickly calmed down. And in 6 months, she lost 40 pounds, bringing her down to 130, which is healthy for her 5-foot-7 frame. Gradually, she allowed herself to go back to eating some sugar, this time in a more controlled manner. These days, she drinks spring water flavored with natural fruits, uses saccharin in her tea, and limits her cookies to just three or four throughout the day.

"If I eat a lot of sugar now, it wipes me out," she says. "So I pretty much stay away from it."

---

*WINNING ACTION*

**Convince yourself that sugar really is bad for you.** *However you choose to vilify sugar, reinforce it by writing it down in a journal, posting it on the refrigerator, or repeating it like a mantra. Whenever you feel a craving coming on, turn to that statement to help yourself stay focused. Reminding yourself that sugar isn't good for you will help you stick with your goals and increase your chances of eliminating sweets from your diet for good.*

---

# HE FOUND DRIED FRUITS TO BE A SWEET REPLACEMENT

Jason Jette used to live on sweets from vending machines. So when he decided to give up sugar in 2000, he learned to satisfy his cravings by snacking on dried fruit.

For years, Jason's diet consisted of Twix candy bars, Dr Pepper soda, and packaged brownies. But being young and athletic, he never gained weight and didn't give his eating habits much thought. "I was raised on meat and potatoes and always ate a lot of candy," says Jason, a 21-year-old food cooperative employee from Albany, New York.

While still in high school, Jason decided to become a vegetarian. Shortly after graduating, he switched to veganism—giving up all animal products, including dairy. He started thinking about giving up sugar, too, when he learned that most manufacturers use animal bone char—charcoal derived from the burning of animal bones—to purify and whiten cane sugar.

He also read that the agricultural runoff from sugarcane farms in Florida was causing pollution in the Everglades and endangering the habitat that supports the plants and wildlife there. "When human beings start to destroy anything that can't be replaced, I have a problem with it," he says.

At the same time, a sugar-free friend told him how much better he felt since giving up refined sugar. In early 2000, Jason stopped eating sugar cold turkey, the same way he quit smoking. "If there's something I really want to do, I have no problem doing it," he says.

To keep cravings at bay, Jason turned to dried fruit. One spear of papaya or a few pieces of apricot was usually enough to tame any cravings for sugar, and Jason learned to always carry some with him. Sometimes, he even makes his own dried fruit with a dehydrator. "The fruit helped relieve my cravings," he says. "And it's great because the sweetness is so concentrated."

Giving up sugar proved Jason's friend right. He lost about 45 pounds from his 6-foot frame, slimming down to 155. As a bonus, he says, "my energy level is definitely higher and more consistent. I just don't tire as quickly. When I ate sugar, my stamina wasn't as high, and I didn't have as much endurance."

Not too long ago, Jason spent the day biking to the border of Vermont, which is about 50 miles from Albany one way. "I left in the morning and returned at sundown," he says. "I don't think I could have done that when I was eating sugar." Now he goes for long-distance rides regularly.

*WINNING ACTION*

**Next time you get a sugar craving, try eating dried fruit.** *These naturally sweetened treats are packed with nutrients and contain enough natural sugar to calm any sweet tooth. The process of drying fruit concentrates all the nutrients, increasing the proportion of minerals and vitamins. By the same token, calories are also concentrated, so don't get carried away with your munching. Be aware that in order to preserve the color, some fruits contain sulfite preservatives, which can create an allergic reaction in some people. Check the ingredient label if you are sensitive to sulfites or if you suffer from asthma.*

# HE BROKE FREE
# WITH SUGAR-FREE GOODS

In 1993, while trying to take off a few pounds, Jim Grubb finally understood what had been wrong with his diet all these years. "I'd always had the feeling that sugar was not good for me," he says. "I began to realize that starches and sugars were indeed contributing to my weight, so I decided to get them out of my life."

Jim, of Scottsdale, Arizona, started paying closer attention to nutrition labels and was amazed at the amount of sugar he ate without realizing it. So he began to steer clear of the supermarket aisle that's land-mined with cookies and candy bars. "We threw out all the cookies in our house and tried to establish not eating sugar as a way of life," he says. "It's hard to discipline yourself when you have a lifetime of that behind you, so once in a while, I eat a Nestlé bar. I used to gobble them, but I quit doing that."

Since he's concerned more about limiting sugar than about cutting out sweet things altogether, Jim and his wife turn to sugar-free substitutes whenever possible. "My wife makes sure to buy sugar-free candies to suck on instead of sugared ones," Jim says. "We even buy sugar-free cough drops. We don't notice a difference between the sugared and sugar-free versions."

He's also been able to find a tasty replacement for his favorite sweet food: ice cream. "At TCBY, I buy a no-fat, no-sugar frozen yogurt, which is much better for me than ice cream," he says. On occasions that call for a dessert, such as having guests over for dinner, Jim serves angel food cake—which, he says, "is fairly innocuous if you must have a sweet" because it's airy and nonfat—and tops it with the "no-sin" yogurt.

Since cutting back on sugar, Jim has lowered his weight from 187 pounds to 175 and kept it there. "Getting along in life requires doing less of what's bad for you and more of what's good," says the 5-foot-10-inch 82-year-old. "I think it was Eisenhower who said, 'The only battles you ever win are battles over yourself.'"

## WINNING ACTION

**Buy sugar-free versions of favorite foods.** *The worst thing about sugar is that it's basically empty calories that provide no nutrients and do nothing more than turn into fat if you don't work them out of your system. Sugar-free foods typically contain fewer calories because the artificial sweeteners they use, like aspartame, acesulfame-K, saccharin, and stevia, contain few or no calories. If you* *can't bear to give up sweet nothings, at least you can choose their sugar-free twins instead.*

## HE WORKED SUGAR OUT OF THE PICTURE

Craig Weintraub knows from experience that offices are loaded with sugar land mines. "When you get in in the morning, the baked goods are waiting for you," says Craig, a 44-year-old resident of Palmer, Pennsylvania. And even though he never considered himself a breakfast person, he'd grab a sugar-laden cinnamon bun when he got to work, starting the day on a sugar high.

Even worse, he says, are the afternoons, "when you get that urge to eat and the only things in the vending machine are candy and high-saturated-fat items." When you have a choice of sugary bars or nothing, the sugar invariably wins. Unfortunately, as Craig points out, "Then you crash later and feel even worse than you did before."

These days, Craig's office offers him a much different environment—but that's only because he's made the effort to stock it with low-sugar snacks. He made the decision to improve his eating habits in December 1999, when he started feeling out of breath after minor physical exertion and was tired after getting 8 hours of sleep. His mother had died of a heart attack, his father of stroke and diabetes. Craig knew that if he didn't make changes, he'd be following in his parents' footsteps.

Those changes started at the office, where Craig spends much of his day. "Until the vending company hears differently from its customers, it's going to stock the machines with candy bars and nacho chips," he says. "If you don't have willpower and you're hungry, naturally you're going to go for something fat and sweet."

A better idea, says Craig, is to stock your desk drawer or office refrigerator with some yogurt, low-fat cottage cheese, or protein bars—something that will fill you up. If you can't get fresh vegetables or an apple or other fruit in your office snack room, bring these things from home.

Sometimes, Craig stashes organic almonds in his desk, and when he feels hungry, he nibbles on five or six of them. "Or I'll have some protein cake," he says. "It looks and tastes like pound cake, but it has 43 grams of protein, 2 grams of fat, and very little sugar."

Craig's treats haven't completely banished his desire for sweets, but he's been able to find plenty of substitutes that keep him from straying back to the vending machines. "There are so many products available that you don't have to eliminate the sweetness at all," he says. "I used to look at people who were in shape and think I could never look the same as them. But I took small steps every day to make smarter food choices and allow time for weight lifting. It's made all the difference."

In fact, in just 18 months, Craig—who stands 5 feet 9 inches—lost 34 pounds of fat and gained 20 pounds of muscle. He now has slightly more than 6 percent body fat and plenty of energy—even on 6 hours of sleep a night.

### WINNING ACTION

**Stock your workplace with better treats.** *It's not like you get candy out of the vending machine for free,* *after all, so why not spend your money on healthier foods at the grocery store? By stockpiling a batch of low-sugar goodies—fresh fruit, sunflower seeds, almonds, whole wheat crackers, protein bars, banana bread—in your desk or office refrigerator, you'll short-circuit that march to the vending machine and give your body more of the nutrients it really needs to get you through the day.*

## SHE CALCULATED THE "EXERCISE COST" OF SUGARY INDULGENCES

An M&M is so tiny. Just one couldn't hurt, could it?

"There is a really good visual exercise for that," says Betsy Lavin, a chiropractor in Wood Lake, Minnesota. "I'd have to walk the length of a football field to burn off the calories from one M&M. When I imagine that, I realize the candy is not worth it to me."

That particular exercise is especially valuable when Betsy is faced with a tempting M&M cookie. "With a dozen M&M's and lots of sugar and fat in it, there's no way I'm going to eat that cookie," Betsy says. "Imagine the workout I'd have to do!"

Betsy, 39, grew up in a country household where dessert was a regular part of the meal. "But we lived on a farm, and we worked really hard," she says. "When I went to chiropractic school, my lifestyle became very sedentary, and I gained weight." At 5 feet 6 inches, she found herself at 226 pounds.

"I ignored it, tried to deny that I was fat," she says. "But I finally got to the point where I realized that it's hypocritical for a person

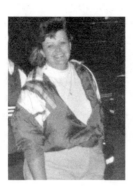

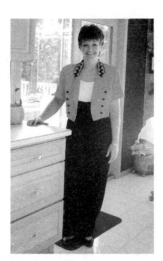

Betsy tapped into her imagination to drop 70 unwanted pounds.

whose business is health and wellness to be 70 pounds overweight."

In May 1997, Betsy joined TOPS Club (Take Off Pounds Sensibly), the oldest nonprofit weight-loss support group in the United States. There she received encouragement from others going through the weight-loss process and learned tricks like the M&M visualization. She also learned to plan ahead with scripted responses when she went out to fast-food restaurants. She rehearsed phrases like "I'll have the chicken sandwich with no mayo, please" and "No fries, thank you." They helped keep her goal of wearing a size 10 in sight.

Within 9 months, Betsy lost 70 pounds. To this day, she maintains her weight at 155.

"I work really hard," Betsy says. "I watch everything I put in my mouth. I keep track of every calorie, and if I choose to eat something, I know I have to work it off—whether by riding my bike to my son's softball games or by doing lots of aerobics and strength training when I can't get out to walk."

Betsy says that sweets in particular were hard to give up. Her mother, who still lives on the farm, would show up at the door in the evening, dessert in hand. "I just had to tell her, 'No, I can't eat it,'" Betsy says. "She doesn't bring it over anymore."

Betsy still uses visualization to avoid tempting sweets. If the call to eat a cookie is too powerful, she breaks it in fourths and eats it throughout the day.

"Cookie or not, the choice is yours," she says. "You are certainly making decisions every day, and it is easy to make the right choice. It all depends on how eager you are for that final reward."

### W I N N I N G   A C T I O N

***Visualize the additional exercise you will have to do to burn off that sweet treat.*** *While the number of calories expended in a particular activity varies, depending on many factors, regular conversation uses between 72 and 84 calories an hour. Riding a lawn mower burns up to 170 calories an hour, vacuuming up to 238 calories, and disco dancing up to 306 calories. Turned around, it takes 1 hour of sawing wood (the outdoors way, not snoring) to work off a piece of pie with ice cream, and 14 solid hours of walking to use enough calories to lose a pound. Get yourself a couple of books: one listing calories in common foods and another showing examples of calories burned during various activities. Spend a few minutes doing the math before you indulge to see whether eating the sweet is worth it.*

## *SHE BATTLED A BEAR CLAW—AND WON*

Don't bother asking Rosanne Paschal her former weight. This vivacious, chatty, 52-year-old Ph.D. won't let on. She *will* tell you that she lost 120 pounds—the equivalent of a whole other person—in 18 months, starting in 1999. And she's kept the weight off her 5-foot frame, a feat she credits to better food choices, exercise, and a few phone calls to her mom.

Rosanne, a radiology educator from Naperville, Illinois, spent 25 years overweight, thanks to a diet that often included cookies, pastries, and the like. In February 1999, already suffering from high blood pressure and high cholesterol and recovering from a bout of kidney stones, she visited an endocrinologist. "He told me I was on the border of diabetes," Rosanne recalls. "He said, 'You're in such bad health, you're lucky if you can walk out of here.'"

Alarmed by the possibility of developing diabetes, she consulted a dietitian, who put her on a strict 1,400-calorie-per-day diet. To stay within her calorie limit, she was advised to eat more complex carbohydrates—choosing a piece of fruit over fruit juice, for example—while limiting sodas, candy, and other foods made with simple sugars.

Within 1 month, Rosanne began losing weight, and within 5 months, she signed on with a personal trainer. "Through 1999, I willed myself not to have any candy or cake at all," she says. But there were times when she was sorely tempted—like the day, several months into her diet, when she bought a prune bear claw.

She never intended to eat it. She just went into a bakery to pick up a carton of milk. When she learned she had to buy a baked good to get the sale price on the milk, she chose a prune bear claw for her husband. Alone in her kitchen with that bear claw, Rosanne's mouth began watering. Temptation loomed, no matter how firm her resolve to resist. "I decided I just wasn't strong enough," says Rosanne. "So I called my mom." Her mother gave her an earful.

"She said, 'Don't you dare!'" recalls Rosanne, chuckling. "She said, 'You've come so far! Go out in the backyard and throw it out for the birds. Don't even put it in the garbage pail! You might go back and get it later.'" Rosanne took heed. She's glad she did. "If you slip up, it can be a real setback for your weight loss," she says. "You may not be able to stop yourself from eating more."

That was the first time Rosanne used the phone to battle a craving. She's done it a few times since. If her mom isn't around, she calls her husband or a friend—anyone who knows how hard she's worked to lose weight. Inevitably, they offer her the support she needs. Only once was she unable to reach someone, leaving her to tackle her craving solo. "I thought about the successful parts of my life and told myself, 'You can do this, too,'" she recalls.

Rosanne has seen tremendous changes in her health since cutting back on sweets. Her body fat, once 50 percent, has dropped to a more reasonable 28 percent. Down to normal, too, are her blood sugar, blood pressure, and cholesterol readings. "I feel so wonderful. I feel energized from eating the right foods," she says. "And I'm not energized from sugar."

## WINNING ACTION

**Phone a friend or relative.** When cravings prove too hot to handle, call for backup support. A close friend, sibling, or parent can help you see beyond the moment of temp-

*tation and remind you that your diet and health are more
important than your sweet tooth. Once you've enlisted
advice, you won't be likely to ignore it.*

# SHE CUTS SUGAR
# FOR HER SON'S SAKE

In spring 1997, Connie Schroer began trying to get pregnant. "I probably weighed somewhere between 230 and 250 pounds back then," she says.

After a year of unsuccessful attempts, she agreed to undergo exploratory surgery in the hope of finding out why she couldn't conceive. Her doctor, an ob/gyn, diagnosed polycystic ovary syndrome (PCOS)—multiple cysts on the ovaries. "He also told me that if I didn't change my eating habits and lose weight, I'd have diabetes by the time I was 40," says Connie, then age 28. "I went home in tears."

While searching the Internet for information on PCOS, Connie found many women with the same condition who were able to get pregnant after losing weight. That convinced Connie to cut out all sugar and refined carbohydrates immediately. This was a tall order considering the bread, pasta, cookies, ice cream, and fast food items Connie was used to eating. "By my postsurgical checkup 2 weeks later, I'd lost 10 pounds," she says. "I was in shock, because I had never been able to lose weight before!"

By sticking with a sugar-free diet, Connie, who lives in New Knoxville, Ohio, lost 37 pounds by the time she got pregnant in September 1998. "You go through withdrawal," she says. "There were several days when I had to have my husband almost sit on me to keep me away from the Little Debbie snack cakes in the cupboard. Once I got through that, I was home free." While she understandably had difficulty keeping to the diet during her pregnancy, by her son's first birthday in June 2000, she was back on the sugar-free wagon and below 200 pounds.

Connie, now 31, has brought her weight down to 171 pounds. Her goal is 145, healthy for her 5-foot-8 frame. She's confident she'll get there. Her motivation is not just her health but her son as well.

"I was a fat kid and endured all the jokes," says Connie. "The last thing in the world I want is to pick my son up from school and have the other children point and call his mommy a fatty. I wouldn't care that they call me that, but I don't want my son to go through it. I want him to be proud of his mother. For me, this is the most powerful motivator in the world."

What's more, says Connie, she's excited about how much she and her son will get to do. "The future holds an active life and a mother who can keep up with her child and bike and hike and do all the things that I would never have been able to do before," she says. "Giving up a moment's pleasure in a bite of cheesecake is well worth the great times we will be having."

## WINNING ACTION

**Be inspired by your kids.** By cutting down on your sugar consumption—and losing the calories that come with sugar—you'll be able to do more with your children on hikes, at the beach, or even when you're just fooling around in the backyard. And since the rate of obesity in children has been rising steadily in the United States, concern for your kids should inspire you to be a good *role model. By eating fewer sweets and maintaining a leaner kitchen, you'll help your children stay as trim as you!*

# *OUT OF SIGHT, OUT OF MIND (AND MOUTH)*

Larry Walker had an ally in his battle to cut out sweets and lose weight: his wife, Patricia.

"My wife has a sweet tooth too," says Larry, 54, of Midlothian, Virginia. "But she keeps sugary stuff out of the house. She doesn't have anything around that would tempt me."

Her strategy worked. Larry, who has diabetes and has had two heart attacks (one in June 1997 and another 11 months later), has lost over 65 pounds. His triglycerides, once an astounding 800, are 134. And his diabetes, with the help of the prescription medicine metformin hydrochloride (Glucophage), is under control.

Larry's bad eating habits were formed years ago, when he was still in diapers. "When I was young, they bribed me with cream doughnuts for potty training," he says. "I still love cream doughnuts. Give me a cream doughnut, and I'll follow you anywhere."

Larry says that before his heart attack, it wasn't unusual for him to eat a dozen doughnuts in 2 days. But the dough rings weren't his only problem. "If it didn't move, I ate it," he says. "And if it did move and it stopped, I might have eaten it anyway!"

He indulged in pastries, pies—and lots of sweetened iced tea. "I made it myself, and it was pretty sweet," Larry says. "I would drink 2 gallons a day."

Then, at the age of 49, Larry suffered his first heart attack. "That really scared me," he says. "I was in combat as a young man, and I wasn't as scared then as I was when I had that heart attack. It surely got my attention."

Larry started eating the way his doctor wanted him to eat. He eliminated sweets—at that time, he was being monitored for type 2 (non-insulin-dependent) diabetes—and started exercising.

"I was really depressed with the second heart attack," he says. "I had worked so hard. My doctor told me that I had done wonderfully for 11 months, but that I had gorged myself for 48 years before that. I needed more time."

As it turned out, he also needed a quadruple bypass. After surgery in June 1998, Larry entered a cardiac rehabilitation program, then gradually resumed his healthy diet and exercise regimen. Five months later, he learned step aerobics and steadily increased his workout levels, wearing a heart rate monitor so he'd know when to slow down.

He no longer eats cream doughnuts. Water has replaced the iced tea. For an incentive when willpower runs low, he visits heart patients—"If you are going to talk about maintaining a healthy lifestyle, you have to look the part"—and makes regular trips to the gym. For 6 to 9 hours a week, he does cardiac kickboxing, group indoor cycling, and step exercises. At 6 feet, he weighs 192 pounds, down from nearly 260.

"Now when I get hungry, I nibble on vegetables," he says. "I have found other things to direct my attention. And I keep focused on what I was. I will never go back that way."

## WINNING ACTION

**Keep sugary foods out of the house.** *Urges to indulge in chocolate or pastries often hit late at night, when going* *to the store is inconvenient. Even if they hit in midday, when a run to the grocery store is reasonable, the trip there may give you time to remember why you don't really want that candy bar. By the same token, make sure that your kitchen is stocked with healthy snacks; fruits, nuts, even whole-grain cereals can divert a craving. And just like your mother told you, never do grocery shopping on an empty stomach. Not only will you spend more than you should, but you will be tempted to buy those snacks that call to you when you are hungry instead of the more sensible food you know you should have.*

## HE EMPTIED HIS POCKETS AND QUIT BUYING SWEETS

For as far back as he can remember, Mark Ziemann had a difficult time saying no to sweets. "When I was in sixth grade, I would eat a whole can of frosting or a whole container of ice cream. I just wouldn't stop," remembers the 41-year-old music teacher from Stockton, California.

Later, in his twenties, his local convenience store seemed to beckon him several times a week. "I found I was stopping either on the way to work or on the way home," he recalls. And what was he buying? "Snickers bars!" he admits. "But I didn't think about the reasons I was doing it. It was usually that I was watching my weight and I would say, 'I haven't eaten today. I need energy.'"

By 1991, Mark realized all those trips to the candy aisle were sabotaging his weight-loss goals. But how could he battle the daily enticement of the convenience store? He decided to simply empty his pockets before he left the house. Without cash, it became impossible for him to jump out of his car for a candy bar.

Using that technique, Mark managed to cut back on his sugar intake for nearly 10 years. But he ate sweets at home, and he was still dogged by cravings. Then, in July 1999, standing 5 feet 8 inches and weighing 226 pounds, he decided to try the Atkins diet—and in the process, give up sugar altogether. Going cold turkey was tough, but Mark says the sugar-fighting tactics he had in place have enabled him to sustain a mostly sugar-free diet since that time.

One of his best strategies is also one of his oldest. "I try not to carry money with me unless I'm going shopping. If I'm just getting into the car to go to work, I don't take cash. It's hard to use an ATM card to buy a candy bar. You'd think about it a lot before you did that," he chuckles.

Mark says he no longer fights sugar cravings. Nevertheless, sometimes when he is home alone watching TV, he begins longing for a snack. What does he do? "I leave the house," he says. He walks down to the pool in his condominium complex or drives to a local bookstore where he can sit and read. He doesn't carry any money with him, so vending machines and snack shops can't tempt him.

Mark dropped 40 pounds in 6 months in 1999. By steering clear of sugar and avoiding temptation whenever possible, he lost another 10 pounds over time, putting him at his present weight of 175.

### WINNING ACTION

**Don't carry cash.** *Has stopping for an after-work treat become a habit you can't break? Empty your wallet on your* *dresser rather than at the convenience store. Both your budget and your waistline will be the better for it. Worried about leaving home penniless? As long as you have either an ATM card or a credit card in your wallet, you'll be covered for emergencies or unexpected purchases. But it's unlikely you'll pull out the cards to pay for the small, sugary items that add up to big trouble for your waistline.*

## *SHE DITCHED THE DOUGHNUTS AND DID THE DISHES*

Amanda Soliday says she just got tired of being overweight. At 46, the 5-foot-4 park maintenance worker estimates she tipped the scales at 194 pounds for about 12 years. As a member of the park's search and rescue team (which tracks down lost hikers), she found her excess weight was making weekly training sessions difficult. So in June 2000, she made a commitment to slim down.

First, she joined Weight Watchers. Then she took a hard look at what she was eating. "I live in a remote place, so sometimes I feel like I'm deprived," explains Amanda, who resides in Grand Teton National Park in Moran, Wyoming. "Sometimes, I would have two candy bars a day."

In fact, treats were part and parcel of rural life for Amanda. She and her coworkers breakfasted regularly on doughnuts and snacked on Amanda's homemade cookies during breaks. What's more, Amanda typically drank a can of sugary soda every day, and whenever she made the hour-long trip to town, she was sure to pick up

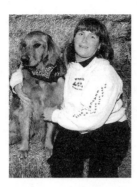

By working through her
cravings, Amanda was able
to lose 57 pounds.

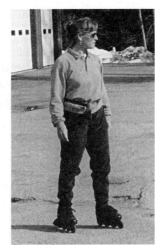

something sweet to munch
on, like Hostess cupcakes or
some candy.

After joining Weight Watchers, Amanda realized she needed
to slice away at her snacking habit. She didn't want to deprive
herself completely, so she agreed to have something sweet once a
week—usually sugar-free chocolate pudding. How did she
manage to steer clear of treats the rest of the time? She worked
through her cravings. Literally. "If you keep busy, your mind
doesn't think about the cravings," Amanda found.

Household chores turned out to be an easy distraction. If she
started longing for a home-baked cookie, she headed to the sink and
washed the dishes. Even that simple task was enough to keep her
from reaching for a snack, Amanda says. Sometimes, when a craving
hit, she took her dog for a nice long walk—she typically walks at
least 3 to 4 miles a day and adds in some mountain climbing in the
warmer months. And even if she wasn't home, she put her strategy
into action. At work, when a box of doughnuts was opened, she

headed out the door. "I'm stationed in a park, so I can always leave and do something else," she says.

In 7 months, Amanda dropped 57 pounds, bringing her down to 137. She's happy with her present weight but wouldn't mind losing another 10 pounds. Amanda admits that fighting initial cravings was tough. Not anymore. "Once you get in the groove of the whole thing, it's easier," she says.

### WINNING ACTION

**Get busy.** *Don't give in to temptation; get out of its way! Doing chores or heading outside for a walk can help you shake off a desire for sweets. Make a list of household tasks that need doing or physical activities you enjoy. Whenever you start aching for a sugary snack, pull out the list. Whatever you do—clean the garage, walk the dog, wash the car—it's bound to take your mind off your craving and leave you feeling good.*

## SHE LIGHTENED UP ON SUGAR BY LIGHTENING UP ON HERSELF

When Amy Jo Van Bodegraven first tried to cut back on sweets, she set some ironclad rules, including a total ban on all sugar. But it wasn't until she loosened up that Amy Jo was able to rein in her cravings and shed some excess weight.

Amy Jo, who's 25 and lives in Whitehall, Pennsylvania, had more than a sweet tooth. She had sugar radar, which sent signals so strong that she'd awaken in the middle of the night for a treat. Among her favorites were chocolate chip cookies, peanut butter, and anything with coconut on it. "If I knew it was in the house, I'd wake up during the night and want it," she says. "I also knew this wasn't normal."

Having gained 15 pounds since college, Amy Jo decided to go on a strict diet that banished all sweets and instead focused on bran cereals and raw fruits and vegetables. She forbade herself to eat in restaurants, cut out all dairy products and red meat, and eliminated pizza, cheeseburgers, and french fries. She also set out to exercise 2 hours a day with the hope of losing 2 pounds a week.

The plan worked—for about 2 weeks at a stretch. "Then I'd be home alone, and I'd go out and buy cookies, crackers, and Doritos," she says, describing a typical binge. "I'd eat half a bag of cookies, half a bag of Doritos—and tell myself I was a bad person. And telling myself I was a bad person only made me want more."

The vicious cycle continued for a year before Amy Jo lightened up in more ways than one. In mid-2000, instead of trying to shed 8 pounds a month, she decided to aim for just 2. She took up weight training and went on a more reasonable diet, one that featured fruits and vegetables in half of all her meals but that also included occasional sweets. "I realized I had to allow myself some sort of sweet or fun food," she says.

She learned to differentiate between cravings for something sweet and the urge to eat a particular food. "If I was in a bad mood, I probably didn't really want the food," she explains. "I just indulged in something sweet to comfort myself." It was these "bad mood" binges that drove Amy Jo's weight gain, she discovered. At these times, she would eat a lot, but the food never made her feel better, even though she was hoping it would.

"On the other hand, if I was in a good mood and had a productive day and wanted a brownie to reward myself, I wasn't eating just to have a pick-me-up," she adds. "So I'd have the brownie, and it was no big deal. I never felt guilty about it afterward or ate a lot at one time. It was simply a treat."

Most important, she stopped judging herself based on what she ate. "I no longer focus on depriving myself," she says. "If I want pizza, I'll just order one. If I want Girl Scout cookies, I set aside 300 calories from another part of my day so I can still enjoy them."

Going easy on herself has worked. Amy Jo lost 8 pounds in the first 2 months and has since lost 2 more. At 5 feet 2 inches, she weighs 114 pounds and rarely craves sweets at all. "I eat so many fruits and vegetables throughout the day that I'm generally full," she says. "If I do crave sweets, it's usually out of boredom. And even then, I might just eat something like an ice cream sandwich. I don't worry about it anymore. I think I have it under control now."

### WINNING ACTION

**Take it easy on yourself.** *Rather than set harsh, unrealistic rules and goals to control your cravings, establish guidelines you can live with, even if it means including an occasional sweet. Also, be sure to stop judging yourself according to the sweets you eat, which will only fuel your cravings if you don't meet your goals. A little self-forgiveness will help you ride out the rough spots and forge ahead in cutting back on sugar.*

# SHE MARKED HER PROGRESS ON THE CALENDAR

Marie Isaac Madison only wanted to pay tribute to a friend. She never expected to end up quitting sugar for good.

"In April 1997, I lost a very good friend of mine from high school in a car accident," says Marie, who lives in Allen Park, Michigan. "She had been a vegetarian since I'd known her, so to honor her life, I decided I would eat vegetarian for a year."

Then in the fall of 1997, Marie's mother learned she had breast cancer. As part of her treatment, she was encouraged to remove dairy foods from her diet. "I joined my mother in eliminating dairy," says Marie.

As she moved toward a completely vegan diet—one that eliminates all animal products—Marie found support in an e-mail pen pal who had been a vegan for decades. "He also abstained from sugar, calling it a drug!" says Marie.

The pen pal suggested Marie read up on sugar's effects on the body, and before long, she was convinced that he was right. "Sugar wasn't any good for me," she says. "So one of my New Year's resolutions for 1998 was to eliminate sugar from my diet." The plan went as follows:

**January:** Eat sweets only on special occasions
**February:** Eat no sweets
**March:** Give up alcohol and sauces with sugar
**April:** Give up refined white flour and pasta
**May:** All sugar will be gone!

As Marie worked toward these monthly goals, she made many changes for both herself and her family. "Before, I kept a stash of chocolate around the house, and I used my monthly celebration as an excuse to binge on sugar," she says. "I don't use that excuse anymore. I also would bake cakes, brownies, and cookies frequently—no more."

Marie stopped picking up candy bars while in line at the grocery store. She converted meals made with white rice and regular spaghetti into dishes with brown rice and whole wheat pasta.

Since becoming a vegetarian, 34-year-old Marie has lost a total of 21 pounds, 7 from sugar reduction alone. The 4-foot-11 computer programmer now weighs 115 pounds. "Yes, I still get sugar cravings, but they're rare," she says. When they do occur, she tries to douse them with sweet fruits like oranges and apples.

"Sometimes, I look back and am amazed at how I used to eat, especially since I had always tried to eat healthy and thought I had achieved it," she says. "But I see that I eat so much healthier now. I feel more in control of my emotions and have more confidence in how I look because I maintain a lower weight. Even my skin glows."

## WINNING ACTION

**Work the sugar out in stages.** *Your sugar-fighting plan doesn't need to be austere. But having some sort of master plan will help guide you toward healthier eating. Maybe your goal for the first month is to drink no more than one soda per day. The month after that, you might cut soda out completely. Or perhaps you'll remove the candy dish from your desk at work. By giving yourself a month to adjust to each change—and not trying to cut out everything at once—you increase your chances of success in the long run.*

# SUGAR HAS NO PLACE
# IN HER PLANS

"I've always known that processed sugar is not my friend, that it has a negative effect on my weight, my metabolism, and my overall health," says Denise Marois-Wolf, of Springfield, Virginia. But until the past few years, she never worried about it that much.

Denise's new outlook came about in several ways. "I started suffering severe anxiety disorder and wasn't able to take my daily walks anymore," she says. "Then I did the AIDS ride in 1997"—a 350-mile ride from Raleigh, North Carolina, to Washington, D.C., over 4 days—"and actually gained weight. I ate too many carbs, too much sugar. I was eating like a teenager.

"Meanwhile, I was entering perimenopause, and I just wasn't burning up calories the way I used to," she continues. "I also took an office job, and my level of activity fell. By 2000, my dress size was heading into the double digits." At 5 feet and 138 pounds, she decided she had to make some changes.

To stop the weight gain, Denise started exercising again on a regular basis, whether walking, swimming, or weight lifting. She also plans to resume karate training, a "great calorie-burner" that she stopped years ago. "When you train hard at anything, you don't want to throw your effort away on sugar," she says.

"When I start to crave sugar, I play little mind games with myself, like going into a nearby department store and drooling over all the beautiful clothes cut for women with skinny hips," adds Denise. "I promise to sew myself a whole new wardrobe with some gorgeous fabric I've bought in Paris or London."

When that's not enough to stop the cravings, Denise thinks of a bigger goal to distract herself, something she can pay attention to other than the call of the sweets. "When your stomach starts to hurt and you start salivating at the thought of something sweet, you have to remind yourself that there are many, many other ways to nurture yourself," she says. "Plan a vacation where you'll be seen in a swimsuit or promise yourself a trip somewhere."

These days, Denise weighs in at 130 pounds—though because she's adding muscle from lifting weights, she knows the scale can be deceiving. A better measure is the fit of her clothes: She's a trim size 8 and nearing an even trimmer size 6. "I'm 50 years old, and I'm feeling pretty darned good about myself," she says.

For those who find themselves in the same shoes she once did, Denise offers the following advice: "Do something that's good for you, that doesn't further detract from your self-respect or your goals. A year from now, either you can be the same—or you can be better."

### W I N N I N G   A C T I O N

***Block sugar cravings by planning for the future.*** *Create a goal for yourself that can be achieved only if you keep yourself away from the sweets. Maybe you want to fit into a new bathing suit that's one size smaller, or you sign up to participate in a walkathon or charity bike race, something that will require stamina and endurance. Each time you push aside sugar, you take an important step toward that goal. Before you know it, you'll have achieved that goal, and you'll be pushing toward the next one.*

# SHE KEPT CUTTING SUGARY FOODS UNTIL NONE WERE LEFT

"I have never been thin," says Serena Edwards, of Port Mansfield, Texas. "As a child, I was obese. At 5 years old, I weighed 96 pounds; by the time I was 8, I was 128 pounds. When I graduated from high school, I was up to 339 pounds." Serena tried a number of weight-loss programs, including fasting and low-fat plans, but they never worked for her.

Now, at age 26, Serena has conquered her weighty past by attacking the one part of her diet that she'd never paid attention to: sugar. "I was a sugar addict," she says. "I could eat a whole bag of fat-free candies in one sitting."

Serena started her no-sugar, low-carbohydrate diet in late 1999. While it hasn't always been a smooth ride, she has stuck to it by adjusting her fat or sugar intake whenever her body seems ready to rebel against losing more weight. "Everyone's body is different," she says. "I've been at this for over 2 years, and I've yet to find any particular thing that works, because my body is constantly changing. Certain things that work one day don't work the next, so I have to keep experimenting to find what's best."

Drinks were one part of Serena's diet evolution. "I no longer drink sugary soda by the liter," she says. And after trying diet sodas, she crossed them off her list as well in favor of water and the occasional iced tea. "If I have that sweet taste, I want more."

Serena also discovered that many sugar-free foods still contain sweeteners that "seem to act like sugar in the body," she says. "I learned that the hard way. A lot of times, even artificial sweeteners trigger responses in my body and make me crave sugar." As a result, she now avoids those foods.

After much experimenting, Serena has reduced her diet to the basics: chicken, beef, pork, fish, vegetables, salads, and a lot of water. While it may sound austere, Serena has been delighted by the results. The 5-foot-9 chef now weighs 160 pounds, down 180 pounds from her top weight.

"Once you get away from the sweet taste of sugar, you don't crave it anymore," she says. "I'm not sure what the future has for me, but I know that I'll be more fit and healthy to face it. My little girl now has a mommy who isn't too tired and fat to play with her and take her places. The weight is coming off slower now, but I didn't gain it all in one night. I've never been this thin, so I'm in no hurry."

### W I N N I N G   A C T I O N

**Keep eliminating sugary foods until your cravings disappear.** *By constantly experimenting with your diet, you should be able to discover what triggers your sugar cravings. Maybe it's soda—even the diet soda that others can drink with impunity. Maybe it's the sweet pickles with lunch or the tomato sauce in your pasta. Whatever the item is, cut it from your diet and see how your eating habits are affected. The goal here isn't necessarily to eliminate all sugar from your life but to make sure that eating sweets is a choice, not a compulsion. It may take you months to find which foods you can eat and which send up a red flag, but it's worth the effort.*

# RESOURCES

## *50 TOP SUGAR SOURCES*

It's been said before in this book, but it bears repeating: You do *not* need to eliminate every last gram of sugar from your diet. That's a good thing, because as you'll discover (if you haven't already), sugar seems to be everywhere, in foods you'd never suspect.

What you want to focus on is *added* sugars—or more precisely, the added sugars in five categories of foods and beverages: nondiet sodas, candy, sweetened baked goods (including cereals), ice cream, and sweetened fruit drinks and iced tea. Just cutting back on these sweets can make a dramatic difference in your total sugar consumption.

The following chart shows you how 50 popular foods and beverages compare in terms of their sugar content per serving. The chart is by no means comprehensive, but it can give you some idea of where you may be overdoing it. For example, 12 ounces of cola contains 39 grams of sugar—just 1 gram shy of the recommended total intake for a 2,000-calorie-a-day diet. And many people drink two or more colas a day!

| Item | Portion | Sugar (g) | Calories |
|---|---|---|---|
| **Sodas and Tonic Water** | | | |
| Cream soda | 12 oz | 49 | 190 |
| Mountain Dew | 12 oz | 46 | 170 |
| Orange soda | 12 oz | 46 | 180 |
| Cola | 12 oz | 39 | 150 |
| Root beer | 12 oz | 39 | 150 |
| Lemon-lime soda | 12 oz | 38 | 150 |
| Ginger ale | 12 oz | 32 | 125 |
| Tonic water | 12 oz | 32 | 125 |
| **Candy** | | | |
| Peanut brittle | ½ cup | 48 | 335 |
| Caramels | 5 (1.8 oz) | 33 | 190 |
| M&M's | 1 pkg. (1.69 oz) | 31 | 235 |
| Butterscotch candies | 5 pieces | 29 | 120 |
| Almond Joy, fun-size | 3 (2.1 oz) | 27 | 280 |
| York Peppermint Pattie | 1 (1.48 oz) | 27 | 165 |
| Licorice Nips | 1 oz | 24 | 120 |
| Chocolate bar | 1 (1.45 oz) | 19 | 205 |
| Marshmallows, miniature | ½ cup | 17 | 200 |
| Jelly ring candies | 5 (1.7 oz) | 4.4 | 190 |
| **Ice Cream and Frozen Confections** | | | |
| Ben & Jerry's Chocolate-Fudge Brownie | ½ cup | 30 | 250 |
| Breyer's Low-Fat Peach Frozen Yogurt | ½ cup | 24 | 125 |

| Item | Portion | Sugar (g) | Calories |
|---|---|---|---|
| Orange sherbet | ½ cup | 24 | 135 |
| Weight Watchers Light Praline Crunch | ½ cup | 21 | 140 |
| Healthy Choice Low-Fat Mint Chocolate Chip | ½ cup | 20 | 120 |
| Chocolate-dipped ice cream cone | 1 avg. | 19 | 185 |
| French vanilla soft serve | ½ cup | 19 | 185 |
| Fudgesicle | 1 (2.5 oz) | 15 | 90 |
| Ice cream sandwich | 1 (3 oz) | 15 | 140 |
| **Baked Goods** | | | |
| Sponge cake | 1 slice (2.8 oz) | 33 | 285 |
| Pumpkin pie | 1 slice (⅛ of 9" pie) | 29 | 315 |
| Pound cake, fat-free | 1 slice (2.8 oz) | 28 | 225 |
| Pound cake, made with butter | 1 slice (2.8 oz) | 24 | 305 |
| Apple cobbler | 1 (3.6 oz) | 23 | 200 |
| Jelly-filled doughnut | 1 (3 oz) | 19 | 290 |
| Blueberry muffin, low-fat | 1 (2 oz) | 19 | 130 |
| Glazed doughnut | 1 (2 oz) | 14 | 240 |
| Fig cookie | 1 | 6.7 | 55 |
| Chocolate sandwich cookie | 1 | 5.0 | 65 |
| **Cereals** | | | |
| Granola, low-fat | 1 cup | 27 | 360 |
| Kellogg's Cracklin' Oat Bran | 1 cup | 21 | 265 |

| Item | Portion | Sugar (g) | Calories |
|------|---------|-----------|----------|
| **Cereals (*cont.*)** | | | |
| Kellogg's Frosted Flakes | 1 cup | 17 | 160 |
| Ralston Purina Crispy Mini Grahams | 1 cup | 17 | 210 |
| Quaker Honey-Nut Toasted Oatmeal | 1 cup | 13 | 190 |
| **Fruit Drinks and Iced Tea** | | | |
| Minute Maid Fruit Punch | 8 oz | 32 | 120 |
| Orange drink, canned | 8 oz | 32 | 125 |
| Grape Fruitopia | 8 oz | 31 | 125 |
| Hi-C Fruit Punch | 8 oz | 26 | 100 |
| Lemonade, from concentrate | 8 oz | 23 | 100 |
| Iced tea, instant | 8 oz | 17 | 70 |
| Cherry Kool-Aid | 8 oz | 16 | 100 |

# INDEX

Underscored page references indicate boxed text and Winning Actions.

## A

Activity. *See also* Exercise
  for avoiding temptation, 224
Alcohol, restricting, 144
Anxiety, exercise for controlling, 126
Appetite, increased sugar and, 27
Artificial sweeteners
  cooking with, 191
  increased appetite and, 27–28
  pros and cons of, 28

## B

Bagels, for reducing sugar cravings, 140–41
Baked goods, sugar in, 4–5, 16, 16
Beer, 144
Bitter foods, for controlling sugar cravings, 47
Blood sugar, 24
Breakfast, importance of, 60, 68–69
B vitamin deficiency, fatigue from, 27

## C

Candy, sugar in, 4, 15–16
Candy bars, snack-size, 173
Carbohydrates, limiting, 67

Cavities, from sugar, 31
Cereals
  fiber in, 73
  sugar in, 4–5, 6, 15, 16
Change, stages of, 155
Chewing, 70–71
Chewing gum, sugarless, 167–68
Children, inspiration from, 217–18
Chocolate, cravings for, 17
Clothes, too-small, as weight-loss reminder, 179
Coffee, eliminating sugar from, 189
Cold turkey, 112
Cookbooks, diabetic, 56
Cravings. *See* Sugar cravings

## D

Deadline, for giving up sugar, 35
Dehydration
  causing sugar cravings, 21
  fatigue from, 27
Desserts
  leftover, giving away, 193
  sweetened with fruit, 195
Diabetes, type 2, sugar and, 30
Diabetic cookbooks, 56
Diet, lifestyle changes vs., 153

237